Survival Guide for Beginners 2021:

The Complete Beginners Guide For Urban And Wilderness Survival In 2021

Leslie Martin

© Copyright 2020 by Leslie Martin. All right reserved.

The work contained herein has been produced with the intent to provide relevant knowledge and information on the topic on the topic described in the title for entertainment purposes only. While the author has gone to every extent to furnish up to date and true information, no claims can be made as to its accuracy or validity as the author has made no claims to be an expert on this topic. Notwithstanding, the reader is asked to do their own research and consult any subject matter experts they deem necessary to ensure the quality and accuracy of the material presented herein.

This statement is legally binding as deemed by the Committee of Publishers Association and the American Bar Association for the territory of the United States. Other jurisdictions may apply their own legal statutes. Any reproduction, transmission or copying of this material contained in this work without the express written consent of the copyright holder shall be deemed as a copyright violation as per the current legislation in force on the date of publishing and subsequent time thereafter. All additional works derived from this material may be claimed by the holder of this copyright.

The data, depictions, events, descriptions and all other information forthwith are considered to be true, fair and accurate unless the work is expressly described as a work of fiction. Regardless of the nature of this work, the Publisher is exempt from any responsibility of actions taken by the reader in conjunction with this work. The Publisher acknowledges that the reader acts of their own accord and releases the author and Publisher of any responsibility for the observance of tips, advice, counsel, strategies and techniques that may be offered in this volume.

TABLE OF CONTENTS

INTRODUCTION 1

CHAPTER 1 *Essential Task List Of Survival* 3

    MINOR EMERGENCY SURVIVAL TASK LIST 4

    MAJOR EMERGENCY SURVIVAL TASK LIST 10

CHAPTER 2 *On-Grid Survival Guide* 15

    SHORT-TERM VS. LONG-TERM ON-GRID SURVIVAL 16

    SECURING SAFETY 17

    SECURING WATER 18

    SECURING FOOD 19

    SECURING FIRE 20

    SECURING SHELTER 21

CHAPTER 3 *Off-Grid Survival Guide* 22

    THE PREPARATION BEFORE THE EMERGENCY 23

    SECURING YOUR FIVE NEEDS FOR SURVIVAL 24

    SETTING YOUR SHORT-TERM SURVIVAL EXPECTATIONS 25

    SETTING YOUR LONG-TERM SURVIVAL EXPECTATIONS 25

CHAPTER 4 *Necessary Survival Materials* 27

    TOOLS FOR WATER 28

    TOOLS FOR SHELTER 28

    TOOLS FOR FIRE 29

    TOOLS FOR FOOD 30

    TOOLS FOR SAFETY 31

    TOOLS FOR TRAVEL 32

CHAPTER 5 *The First Essential: Water* 34

    Locating and Accessing Water...35

    Purifying and Storing Water..37

    Building Your Camp Near a Body of Water...38

    Securing Long-Term Access to Water 40

CHAPTER 6 *The Second Essential: Shelter*..**43**

    Where to Build Your Shelter...44

    Short Term Shelter Solutions 47

    Long-Term Shelter Solutions 48

CHAPTER 7 *The Third Essential: Fire* **53**

    Where to Build Your Fire..54

    Building a Birds Nest...55

    Fire for Heat...57

        Teepee Fire Lay *58*

        Lean-to Fire Lay..*59*

        Log Cabin Fire Lay *60*

        Long Burning Fire Lay *61*

        Dakota Fire Pit *62*

    Fire for Cooking..*63*

        Pyramid Fire Lay *63*

        Star Fire With a Cooking Arm *64*

CHAPTER 8 *The Fourth Essential: Food* **66**

    Types of Food to Eat in the Wilderness...67

    Foraging for Vegetation 68

    Hunting, Trapping, and Fishing 70

    Butchering Small to Medium Game...72

    Butchering Birds 74

    Butchering Fish and Reptiles 76

    Cleaning and Cooking Wild-Caught Meat 77

    Properly Storing Food 78

    Long-Term Gardening Solutions 80

CHAPTER 9 *The Fifth Essential: Safety* **82**

    Protecting Yourself From Predators 84

    Keeping Yourself and Your Camp Hygienic 86

    First Aid Skills You Need to Know 90

        Treating Burns *90*

        Dressing Wounds *91*

        Setting Broken Bones *92*

        Dealing With Illness *94*

    Foraging for Medicinal Plants 95

CHAPTER 10 *The Great Escape* **96**

    Escaping Minor Emergencies 97

    Escaping Major Emergencies 98

CHAPTER 11 *The Unspoken Essential Of Survival* **101**

    The Biggest Danger Lurking At Two AM 102

    Keeping Yourself on Track for Survival 104

CHAPTER 12 *Getting Help When Needed* **106**

    When Is the Right Time to Call? 107

    Who Is the Right Person to Call? 109

    How Can You Prepare to Be Rescued? 111

    Is There Ever a Time When You Should Not Call? 112

CONCLUSION **114**

INTRODUCTION

Whether we like it or not, the affluent societies we have built for ourselves are not always as reliable as we need them to be. Our communities are made to be efficient. They were designed for everyday life in a modern world, so long as everyday life does not include any form of disaster that disrupts the system. The minute one small disaster strikes, though, the entire system can be thrown off course, and anywhere from hundreds to billions of people can be affected by the derailing of the system. This means that, despite how well it works on a good day, the system is unreliable, and you should *always* have a backup plan for when the system fails.

Backup plans can range from simple adjustments you can make to your everyday life to get through disruptions to your usual system and elaborate ideas for how you will escape and survive without any access to the modern system. And before you think, "I don't need something that elaborate!" I encourage you to think again. Natural disasters are increasingly common, with devastating fires, hurricanes, tornadoes, earthquakes, and even pandemics coming through and causing destruction for the populations they impact. In some cases, that destruction can be devastating and can lead to secondary injury, illness, or even death as people find themselves unable to access necessary resources like food, water, or shelter, or they become injured or killed by a damaged environment.

Knowing how to escape a dangerous situation and survive, no matter what the circumstances, is an important part of staying alive. As efficient as our system may be, if it fails, you must know how to survive on your own. With so many disasters that strike our society every year, you never know when one might strike you.

Learning how to survive is not nearly as challenging as you might think, though it does require some basic understanding of what you need to survive, and how you can safely acquire these resources. Clear guidance, combined with common sense and your built-in instincts will help you survive anything that might come your way.

If you are ready to discover how you can survive anything, let's begin.

CHAPTER 1

Essential Task List Of Survival

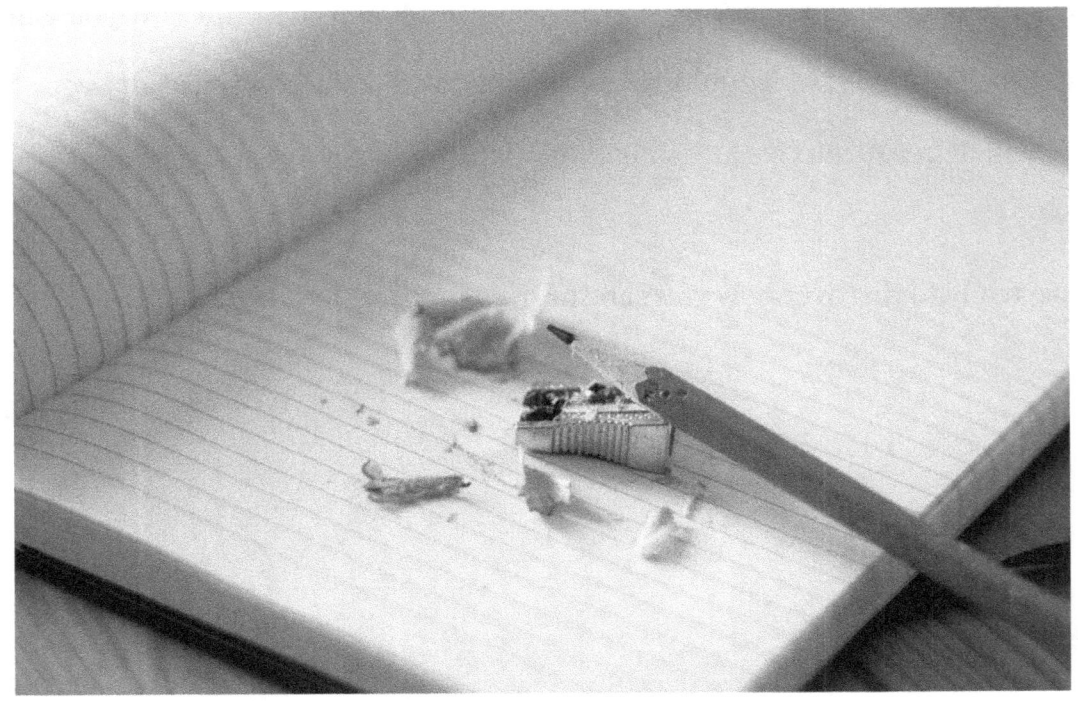

Surviving any situation requires you to know the five requirements of survival, and how you can safely secure those resources. Those who have never survived on their own must understand the importance of safely acquiring necessary resources without expending too much energy. In any survival situation, even minor ones, preserving energy and doing things in a logical manner is the best practice for securing your survival.

The essential task list of survival looks different depending on whether you are in a minor survival situation or a major disaster. In a small survival situation, you do not evacuate the premises so that you will be securing your survival from the comfort of your own home. In an extreme survival situation, you are required to evacuate the premises, so you will need to secure all of these things away from home, possibly in an off-grid situation. At home, emergencies can be classified as minor survivalist emergencies, whereas off-grid survival situations are major emergencies. If you find yourself away from home, but not in need of off-grid survival, you will want to select the survival practices that best fit your individual situation so you can survive in those unique circumstances.

No matter what your circumstances are, to secure your survival, you will require water, shelter, fire, food, and safety. The order in which you acquire these will depend on what stage you are in the unfolding emergency.

Minor Emergency Survival Task List

A minor emergency could be anything from an injury sustained at home, to a house fire, or other similar emergencies. Power outages, storms that make travel dangerous (but that do not affect your ability to stay home,) and other similar events are also minor emergencies. As the crisis is unfolding, you are in an active state of emergency. All minor emergencies, however, are usually isolated quickly, and you can move into a state of recovery rapidly. The exception may be in the instance of storms, such as winter storms, where you are unable to leave your home, so you must stay there. In these scenarios, you cannot guarantee when they will end, though the recovery from these storms is usually relatively quick and does not require evacuation.

If you find yourself in one of these situations, your task list for survival includes: secure safety, water, food, fire, and shelter, and get help.

Task #1: Secure Safety

Securing your safety is paramount in a situation where a minor emergency is unfolding. These emergencies can pose threats to your immediate safety, and if they are not mitigated, you could find the crisis growing more significant and more devastating by the minute. For example, if your house is on fire and you do not seek safety first, you run the risk of being burnt to death.

To effectively secure your safety, you need to ensure that you are aware of what the dangers are and who is around you so you can aid them in achieving their safety, too. However, you must never make the mistake of ensuring their safety *first*. If you are not safe, you will not be able to guarantee the safety of someone else. Often, in a state of panic, individuals will risk their safety to save someone else, only to put themselves in a dangerous situation where they are now both in need of being rescued by someone else. Sadly, this leads to many deaths. For example, if your friend were drowning in fast-moving water, it would not be safe for you to jump in to save them because rather than being able to save them, you, too, would begin drowning in fast moving water. It is extremely challenging to put your own safety above others' at times, but if you do not, you may find yourself also becoming extremely injured or even killed in a failed rescue mission.

To secure your safety, you must look at your surroundings, make a quick assessment of how safe you are in them, and then move to safer surroundings. For example, if you are in a burning house, it is evident that you are not safe, so you must immediately remove yourself from your surroundings. If you can bring your loved ones with you as you get out, do it. Once you are outside, you have reached safety and completed task number one.

Many minor emergencies require escaping a dangerous situation or calling for help to escape a hazardous situation. Some, however, may require you to stay in to avoid a dangerous situation. For example, in extreme winter storms, you may need to shut yourself in your house to protect yourself. In this case, your means of securing safety would be to ensure that all windows and doors are closed and that you have a generator to help you power your house through a possible power outage.

Task #2: Secure Water

Humans cannot survive longer than three to four days without water. When you are panicked, it may be the last thing you are thinking about, but you must stay hydrated if you want to remain healthy and alive. Getting access to clean, safe drinking water as soon as possible is an essential task. Being able to sip on water as you navigate a crisis, or the aftermath of one ensures you do not begin to suffer dehydration, and the many side effects dehydration brings with it. Realize that while you can survive three to four days without water, you will begin to deal with the symptoms of dehydration much sooner. This includes weakness, fatigue, dizziness, headaches, and other symptoms that can make survival much more challenging.

In minor emergencies, the best way to secure water is to already have water on hand. In your house, you likely already have access to tap water, and you may also have drinking water in your fridge. In case these resources run out or are not safe to consume in an emergency, it is also helpful to have bottled water or five-gallon jugs of water with a water dispenser. You will need three to four days' worth of water for every person in your house, including pets, in case of an emergency. You will need at least 3 liters of drinking water per person and animal in your family. You should also have water available for other purposes, such as cleaning, sterilizing your environment, or bathing. This means if you have a family of four plus one dog and one cat, you will need 18 liters of drinking water, plus about 40 to 60 liters of water for other uses such as cleaning. It may sound like a lot, but the average human uses about 80 to 100 gallons of water per day, between bathing, flushing the toilet, washing their hands and brushing their teeth, doing the dishes, and engaging in other water-related activities. Reduce your consumption by using fewer flushes, sharing bathwater, and using wash basins rather than running water, as these will all conserve water.

Task #3: Secure Food

The third task you must secure is food. Humans can survive up to three weeks without food, but the longer you go, the more symptoms you will endure, which will make securing and consuming food far more challenging. In a minor emergency, having access to smaller food items is a great way to ensure you provide yourself with everything you need to stay well-nourished. Having a well-stocked pantry, fridge, and freezer helps, too.

It is advised that you keep two to four weeks' worth of food in your home. You can also keep snack bars, trail mix, beef jerky, and other small, non-perishable, nutrient-dense snacks in emergency locations, such as in your car, to ensure proper nutrition during dangerous situations. You would be surprised how hungry you get within minutes or hours of moving out of an active state of emergency and into the recovery phase. Getting nutrients into your body helps you recover from the intense energy demands that the emergency itself placed on your body.

Task #4: Secure Fire

Securing fire may or may not be necessary in minor emergencies. In something isolated, like an injury, fire is likely completely unnecessary. In something such as a power outage, though, securing fire is important. Fire is used for heat to keep your core temperature stable, as well as for cooking. In minor emergencies, replace open fires with electricity, gas ovens, or propane-fueled barbecues for cooking. Insulated clothes and blankets can be used to maintain a proper body temperature. If you are out of electricity and do not have access to a safe fuel source, you can also start a small fire in a homemade pit in your backyard to help you stay warm and cook food with.

Inside of your home, the best way to keep yourself warm is to light candles, pile as many blankets together as you can, and wear warm woolen clothes that are designed to keep you warm. If you are in an extreme situation and cannot get warm, wear a thin layer of clothes, or no clothes, under a blanket with other people so your body temperature can work together to help heat each other up.

Task #5: Secure Shelter

In most minor emergencies, you can stay in your home or somewhere close to home. For example, in the event of a flood or fire, you may have to leave your home, but your town would be perfectly safe for you to stay in. The emergency you are in will decide what needs to be done to protect your shelter in that emergency.

If you are able to stay inside of your house, securing shelter means ensuring that your shelter is safe for you to stay in. This could mean locking doors, or closing and locking windows. You might also need to secure outdoor furniture, so it doesn't blow around and cause harm. If you are in the middle of a winter storm, you may need to close off the doors to the main room in your home, cover the bottom of those doors with towels to prevent heat from escaping, and focus on heating that primary area of your house. The entire key is to ensure that the space you are surviving in is capable of keeping you protected from the elements while giving you adequate space to fulfill your other four basic needs.

Task #6: Get Help

Finally, if you are in an emergency, the minute everything is stabilized, you may need to call for help. Unless it is a minor injury or something else that is relatively small and can be secured at home, without additional help, you will need to be prepared to call for assistance with getting your situation remedied.

A vital step to take *before* you ever reach the point where you need to get help is to have the contact information for anyone who may assist you through any emergency present and easy-to-access at all times. A list on the fridge, for example, is a great way to have these numbers available. Include the local emergency number, authorities, doctors and dentist numbers, poison control, and other essential emergency numbers on your list. You should also include numbers for your personal identification and your health insurance policy, dates of birth, in case any of this is required in an emergency phone call.

Major Emergency Survival Task List

If you are in a major emergency survival situation, the approach is going to be much different. In major emergencies, you can be driven out of your home with very little time to prepare, and you may need to survive in the wilderness for an extended period of time. Knowing how to protect yourself and your family in these types of emergencies is important. It is also where many people are largely unprepared and find themselves making serious mistakes that can lead to injury, illness, or even death. We will cover all of these tasks in far greater detail later in this book, but for now, you need to know what these tasks are and what order they fall in.

Task #1: Secure Water

The first task you must fulfill immediately upon escaping a dangerous situation is securing water. You can only survive three to four days without water, but after one day, you can start experiencing serious side effects from not being hydrated enough. Since it can take some time to access and purify water for drinking in the wilderness, you need to make it your number one priority to find some. This way, if it takes you a day or more to find any water sources, you have enough time actually to find them before dehydration ultimately proves fatal.

Another benefit of securing water first, aside from it saving your life, is that you know where the water is and can build your camp near the water source so that it is easy for you to access that water source continually.

Task #2: Secure Shelter

Securing shelter should always be your second move after obtaining water. Your shelter should be close enough to water so that it is easy to access, but not so close that the water poses a threat itself. Your goal with shelter in off-grid survivalist situations is to create a shelter that maintains your core temperature, keeps you comfortable, and provides you with safety from the elements. This means you will need to build it away from widowmakers, or environmental dangers that can instantly kill you if they are triggered, and in such a way that fulfills your needs for shelter.

If you were able to bring supplies with you, a shelter can easily be built out of tarps and rope. If you were not, you will have to use elements of the environment to build your shelter. The environment features many resources you can use to create high-quality, lasting shelter in any situation. For example, trees, branches, mud, leaves, stones, and even snow can be used to create a shelter for yourself, depending on what situation you are in. As long as it can protect you from the elements and provide a safe space for you to stay warm in, it is plenty for your shelter.

Task #3: Secure Fire

After you have secured your shelter, you need to secure fire. Fire is used in an abundance of ways in off-grid survival situations. Fire provides warmth, a means for cooking, and a way to sterilize your tools and yourself. There are many reasons you will use fire in a survival situation, so be prepared to know how to create adequate fire lays for any circumstance. In the wilderness, there are many options for the types of fires you can build. You will need to know how to build a variety of fires, as they will all support you with keeping yourself safe. Specific fire lays can be used to keep you warm overnight, heat your camp for a few hours, cook, or alert others to your whereabouts through smoke signals. Each fire lay is also designed to prevent your fire from growing out of control to ensure you do not accidentally start a forest fire.

Task #4: Secure Food

If you have time on the day of your arrival in your survivalist location, you will want to secure food. If it is later in the day or into the evening, though, you will want to wait as food can take a while to secure. Starting on day two, focus all your efforts on securing food as you will need as many calories as possible to sustain yourself in the wilderness. You will need a variety of foraged vegetation and meat to keep yourself going, especially in the wilderness, as the protein will be important for keeping your energy up and allowing you to survive the pressure being placed on your body.

With securing food, you will also need to secure a means for cooking and preserving that food. In the wilderness, this requires additional measures you must take to prevent predators from hunting you based on the scents you are creating through the foods you are cooking. Especially as you kill, cook, and store meat, you will be at risk of attracting predators who may try to steal your meat from you. Proper safety measures will ensure you can accomplish all of this without harming yourself or losing your bounty to another predator.

Task #5: Secure Safety

Safety is paramount in survivalist situations, especially when you are off-grid. Off-grid, you do not have access to things like doctors, emergency responders, police, firefighters, or anyone else who can help you out of a dangerous situation. You must place safety first so you can prevent hazardous situations from arising, hopefully meaning you never actually need emergency support in your survivalist situation. If you do, keep safety kits available to help you deal with any emergencies you may face. These emergency kits ensure you can navigate any situation safely and successfully.

Task #6: Get Help

After you have secured your survival, you need to get help. This might include traveling into cell service, finding your way back to a major civilization where someone can help you, or even using flares or smoke signals to indicate where you are if a search and rescue team is searching for you. Getting help is important, as help is how you will be able to ultimately get yourself out of this situation and back into a safe civilized location.

There are, however, times where you may not be able to call for help. For example, if you are escaping a police state or a major emergency like a pandemic, it may not be feasible for you to call for help. Unfortunately, people often find themselves in situations where they cannot or should not rely on the help that would otherwise be available to them. In these scenarios, those who may claim to help you might actually cause more harm than they would solve. In this case, you would omit calling for help and instead begin focusing on tasks that will set you up for long-term survival.

CHAPTER 2

On-Grid Survival Guide

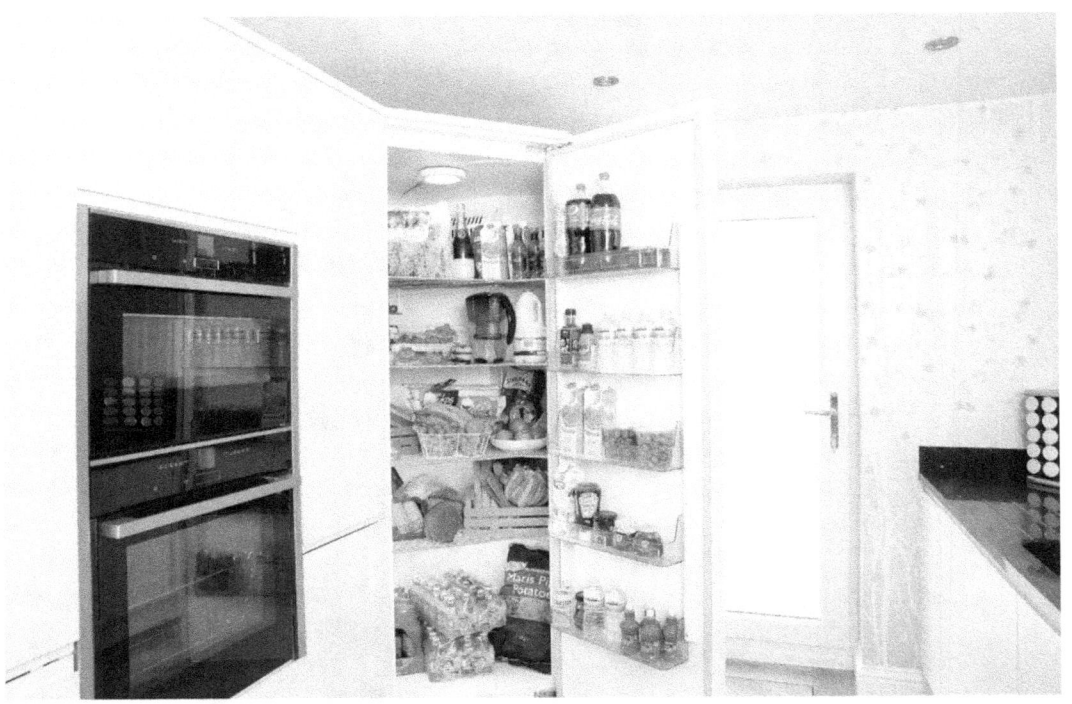

The on-grid survival guide is undoubtedly the more comfortable survival guide to follow. On-grid, many tools exist to help you meet your survival needs. You should leverage them in every way possible, as they will minimize the amount of energy you have to exert while also keeping your habits as close to normal as possible. If you can, lean on corporate resources to stock yourself up with everything you need to survive. All you need to do, then, is know how to do this efficiently and effectively to secure your survival.

One thing I cannot stress enough is the importance of knowing that you are responsible for your own survival. In an emergency, you may find yourself wanting to wait for the government or public health officials to direct you on what to do and where to go. The problem with this is that it could take hours, days, or even weeks for them to organize everything and get enough resources to sustain everyone effectively. In the meantime, you could be floundering as you have not been able to access the resources you need. While relying on this system to get more resources is helpful, it is important that you have your own plan in place so that you are not waiting for someone else to promise you your safety. Instead, you can take it into your own hands and secure your safety and the safety of your family, which will result in your successful survival.

Short-Term VS. Long-Term On-Grid Survival

Short-term on-grid survival and long-term on-grid survival both look the same; however, you will need more supplies for long-term survival than you will for short-term survival. Most on-grid survival situations will be short-term. Some, however, may be long-term. For example, amid the pandemic of 2020, many were forced to self-isolate or stay home for extended periods without direct and consistent access to necessary resources, such as grocery stores or their general health practitioners. Another example of long-term on-grid survival would be if you lived in a place where winters were severe, and power could be out for days or even weeks on end, or if the harsh weather eliminated your ability to access resources such as the grocery store.

For long-term survival situations, you need to have an abundance of water, food, and heat sources available at a moment's notice, or the ability to quickly access it if you do not have any readily available. You also need to have the ability to defend yourself, administer basic health-care needs if necessary, and secure your shelter. Ideally, you should have enough to protect yourself for up to one month. However, you may prefer to have more if you will be in a situation where you know accessing resources will be nearly impossible for extended periods.

Securing Safety

Securing your safety on-grid starts with assessing your environment, identifying possible hazards, and protecting yourself from any impending dangers. In obvious cases, such as during a fire or flood, this means escaping the affected building and getting yourself into a safe space. In less obvious situations, though, this requires more extensive care and attention.

In any environment, there can be a wide number of dangers threatening yourself or your family. Complete an assessment of your environment by quickly studying everything for obvious risks, then scanning from the ground up since most hazards are at ground-level. In your home, this could include stoves, electric outlets, fallen furniture, or other common household hazards. Outside, this might include power lines, traffic, fallen trees, weather, or other landscape or natural hazards. Always be aware of what the likely dangers are in your area, as this allows you to scan in an educated manner and avoid accidental illness, injury, or death.

Be highly aware of anything that could be classified as a widowmaker. Widowmakers are not always apparent at first, but they do have the power to instantly injure or kill a person who came into contact with them. For example, a fallen powerline, broken gas lines, or exposure to chemicals are incredibly unsafe. If you suspect there may be something dangerous in your environment, rectify it, or remove yourself from the situation immediately. Hazards can rapidly turn into actual emergencies without any warning. It is better to remove yourself and your family from the area than to hope it will not become a hazard and find out later that you were wrong. When in doubt, never take a risk that comes with a possible consequence that you would not want to face.

As soon as you have assessed your situation, you need to either remove safety hazards or take necessary measures to remove yourself from the vicinity of those dangers if they are not able to be fixed safely. Safely is the keyword here, as you should never attempt to resolve a hazard by yourself if you are not confident that you can do it by yourself, and sure that you have the necessary tools to do it yourself. If you lack the necessary tools or the know-how, you need to wait for someone more experienced to resolve the safety hazard and instead focus on keeping yourself away from it so it cannot pose a threat to your safety or livelihood. This may mean leaving a certain area, leaving a building altogether, or otherwise moving somewhere safer so that you are no longer at risk of being injured or killed by that hazard.

Securing Water

The easiest way to secure water in an on-grid survival situation is to turn on your tap. In most minor emergencies, accessing water from your taps is still possible. You could then drink it, or run it through a purifying system you already have on hand if you live in a location where water purifiers are needed. If accessing tap water was not possible, though, such as if your water was turned off, a line busted, and you could not receive water through the lines, or your water was contaminated, the next best thing is to buy water.

Water bottles and five-gallon jugs of water are the best way to go, as they ensure you have enough water to get through an emergency. If you are unable to source any, you can also collect rainwater, water from a natural body of water, or uncontaminated snow, and purify it. It is vital that you purify this water properly, however, as they are all likely to have contaminants in them, especially if you are in an urban environment with a high-density population. These areas are known for being highly polluted, which makes them a threat to your health.

Securing Food

Like with securing water, securing food in an on-grid survival setting should be as easy as going to the grocery store and getting some, ideally, you should have at least two weeks to one month's worth of food in your pantry at any given time so that you have plenty to get you through in case accessing the grocery store becomes challenging. If you run out of food at home, you may be able to rely on a local charitable organization to provide you with food until you can secure more. However, some emergencies may lead to you being unable to secure food from these sources.

If you cannot secure food from the grocery store or a local organization, the best thing you can do is turn to fishing or trapping. Fishing is generally legal in most places, while trapping may or may not be legal, depending on where you are. You may need permits to do either activity, though. Avoid hunting in cities or townships, as it would be easy for you to accidentally hurt another person, rather than the animal you were targeting, and that would be devastating. Further, it could bring with it major charges and prison time, which would make an emergency even more devastating for everyone involved.

Securing Fire

Securing fire benefits three primary things associated with your survival. Fire maintains your core temperature, helps you cook, and allows you to adequately sterilize things in your environment through either smoke or boiling water. In an urban environment, actual fire may not be necessary as you may be able to secure these three things in different ways. For example, if you have access to electricity, a stove or barbecue, and washing agents, you should not need to have a fire to secure these elements. If, however, you cannot access electricity, a stove, or a barbecue, you may need to improvise.

The order of improvising should be as follows: if you cannot rely on electricity from your main power source, turn on a generator. If you cannot rely on a generator, turn to a fuel source like propane barbecues or coal-based barbecues. If you cannot rely on a barbecue, turn to candles and fire pits or fireplaces. You can also use warm clothes and blankets to keep your space warm. For cooking, you may be able to eat food items that you can get from the grocery store that does not require cooking, such as cereal, granola bars, beef jerky, fruits and vegetables, bread, and other items that do not need to be cooked. For sterilizing, you can always use cleaning agents such as soap or cleaning products to keep your environment sterile and healthy.

Securing Shelter

Securing shelter should be the easiest thing to do in a minor emergency where you are able to remain on-grid. In most emergencies, even long-term emergencies, you should be able to stay safe inside your home. Ideally, your home should have everything a shelter needs for you to remain safe and secure throughout the emergency. If your home is not an option, you can always stay with a family member or a friend. If that is not an option, you can look into emergency shelters and housing facilities put on by your city, as these locations can often provide you a place to stay until you are able to return to your own home.

CHAPTER 3

Off-Grid Survival Guide

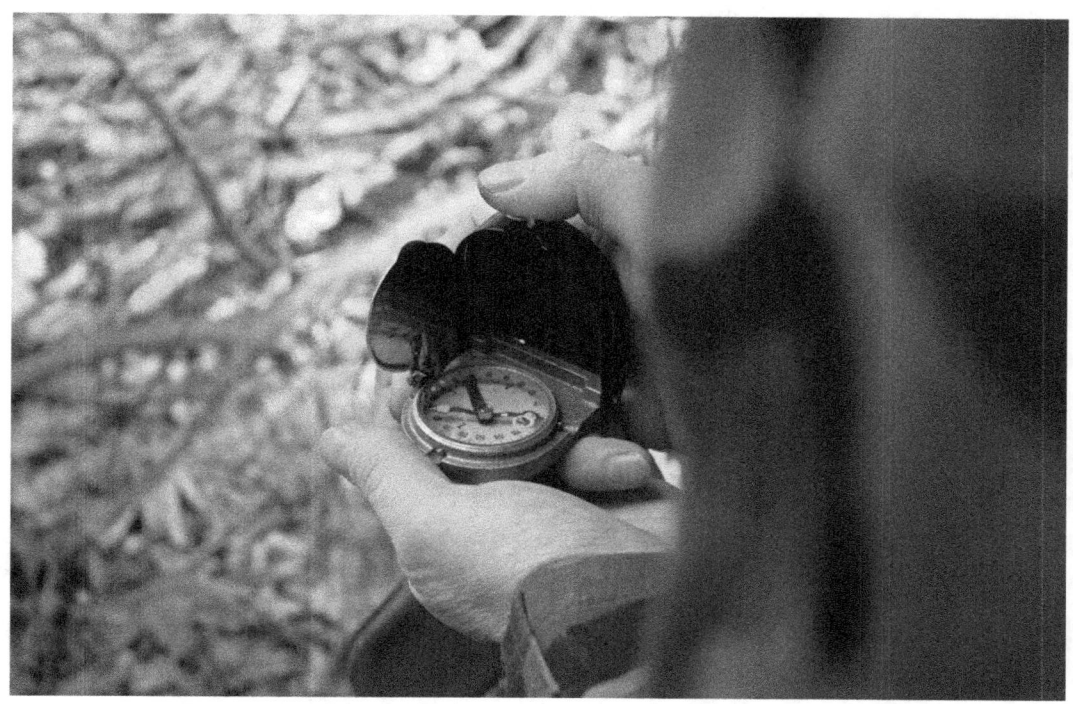

Off-grid survival is far more challenging, requires more energy and effort on your behalf, and takes preparation and know-how. If you have never had to survive off-grid, you likely cannot imagine the amount of work and energy it requires for you to be able to preserve your life in an off-grid environment. Despite how much work it takes, you will be pleased to know that in survival situations, your body is designed with all of the chemicals and hormones you require to stay alert, navigate dangers, and keep yourself going through any problems you face. Still, you need to know what to do and how to do it so that all of your energy and enthusiasm can be applied toward something that will actually turn results.

Surviving off-grid requires far more than I can put in one chapter, so we are first going to discuss what needs to be done for you to survive off-grid. Then, we will discuss all of these measures in far greater detail, complete with tutorials and step-by-step instructions, in later chapters. This way, your mind is organized and ready to receive this knowledge, and you receive the step-by-step guidance you need to put it to work.

The Preparation Before the Emergency

Preparing for an emergency before one actually strikes is the most valuable thing you can do for yourself. Do not fail to prepare because you believe you would never face an emergency, because then when you do, you will not be prepared. Have everything ready so that if something does go wrong, you are prepared for that situation. Many people mistakenly believe that it cannot happen to them, but the reality is that minor and major emergencies alike can strike anyone at any time. None of us are exempt from the dangers lurking in everyday life. Preparation ensures that you have everything you need to survive any one of those dangers, should they strike.

To prepare for your emergency, you need to have the necessary tools and resources readily available, as well as knowledge on how to use those tools and support if need be. This includes having adequate supplies for water, shelter, fire, food, and safety on hand at all times, and knowing exactly how to use all of those tools to get the most out of them. The better you are at preparing, the more ready you will be in the event of an emergency.

Your preparation will come in two parts. The first will include preparing your tools. Your tools will all be bought, gathered, and stored in grab N go bags or G'nG bags, which are designed to make it easy for you to quickly grab all of the necessary tools and evacuate if need be. These should be ready even for minor emergencies that occur at your home, as they will be full of every tool you need to navigate those emergencies. You will also want to have money set aside. If you do find that you need money to navigate a more significant crisis. This way, if you are unable to work for an extended period of time, you do not go bankrupt trying to afford life in the meantime.

Aside from preparing your tools, educate yourself on how they work and when to use them. You should also be trained on how to observe wear and tear, damage, or expiration signs on the tools so that you can replace them. You will want to replace tools as needed in your emergency kit, even if they are going unused, to ensure you have new, useable tools in the event of an emergency.

Securing Your Five Needs for Survival

Preparation is all you will need unless an emergency arises. In the event that an emergency arises, you need to escape your environment and secure your five needs for survival, or your water, shelter, fire, food, and safety. Escaping should be seen as an essential safety measure in your first five, as remaining in an area that has an active emergency is highly dangerous and can lead to injury, illness, or death. We will go into far greater detail on your five needs for survival and how to practically secure each one, as well as how to escape to a safer environment, later.

Setting Your Short-Term Survival Expectations

Your short-term expectations in the wilderness should include having everything you need to get through a few days until help can get to you and bring you to safety, or until it is safe for you to return home. You will likely live in a shelter made of tarps and ground cloths, eat whatever food you were able to deliver with you, and possibly fish or forage for some additional food and drink through whatever water you were able to bring. Depending on your circumstance, you may need to locate and purify water, too. Building fire should also be comfortable enough with whatever fuel sources you brought with you.

Aside from the emergency aspect and the stress and trauma, it can bring with it, surviving in the wilderness for a few days is not unlike taking a camping trip. Although it was not a planned camping trip, and it certainly will not feel relaxing based on the circumstances, the same skills are required, and the same expectations around what it takes to survive will fit this situation, too.

Setting Your Long-Term Survival Expectations

Long-term survival expectations are far more challenging to set, though they are essential as knowing what to expect helps you prepare and endure that situation if you find yourself in it. In a long-term situation, you need to be ready to create more elaborate accommodations to support your survival. Tarp tents and fishing and foraging are unlikely to be enough in this situation. As well, you will likely not want to have to go fill and purify your canteen of water several times a day, every single day. You need to be ready to set yourself up with an elaborate living condition that can sustain you for as long as you need.

Your shelter in long-term survival situations will likely be made of wood, branches, brush, leaves, clay, dirt, and other findings that you can use from the environment to create a warm and comfortable dwelling that keeps you safe from the elements. You will also likely set up a more efficient cooking camp, proper storage measures for your food, and a place where you can gather and store water so that you do not have to fetch it so often. Long-term storage of wood for your fire, as well as tools for preserving your safety, are important. Eventually, predators will come to know where you are and may become more curious about you and what is going on, and you will need to protect yourself from those predators. As far as food goes, hunting and trapping will be useful in long-term survival situations, as well as gardening.

CHAPTER 4

Necessary Survival Materials

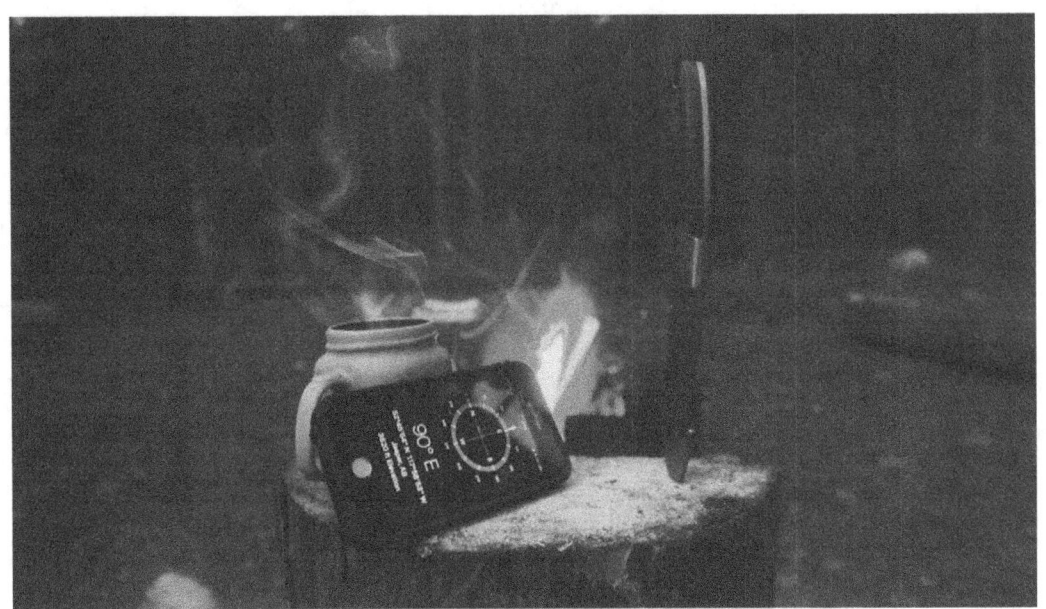

Since preparation is key to success in surviving any situation, you need to ensure that you are prepared at all times. Preparing for survival means having the right materials on hand so that you can navigate any situation with adequate tools. While many tools can be made in the bush, it is often easier to have your own that were made to fulfill specific needs, as they will be more effective and will result in better outcomes. The tools you need will cover everything that has to be done in the wilderness, ranging from traveling to get there or traveling through the wilderness, to securing water, shelter, fire, food, and safety.

In addition to gathering the necessary tools, you need to keep them neatly organized in G'n'G bags so they can quickly be grabbed during an emergency evacuation. This way, you are not scrambling to find all of your tools and put them together in the event that something goes wrong. You also need to review your materials on a regular basis to ensure that they are working, that they still meet current safety standards, and that they have not expired or otherwise sustained damage that makes them unusable.

Tools for Water

For water, you need tools that will allow you to carry and store it, as well as tools that will allow you to purify it.

- Water bottles and storage containers
- Cups
- Water purifying containers
- Water purifying drops

Tools for Shelter

For shelter, you need tools that will enable you to build a well-designed camp. Your shelter will need to be able to protect you from all of the elements, while also offering comfort. You want a shelter that will be easy to design, too, so you are not wasting any energy or frustration over building a shelter for yourself and anyone who is staying at the camp with you.

- Rope and cordage

- Tarps and tarp tents
- Polypropylene
- Silnylon
- Canvas
- Oilcloth
- Ground pads
- Browse bags
- Emergency thermal blankets
- Hammock
- Sleeping bags
- Military modular sleeping system
- Wool blankets
- Saw

Tools for Fire

For fire, you will need devices that will allow you to start a fire, as well as fuel for those devices. You may also need fuel for the fire itself if you are having a hard time getting your fire going.

- Lighters
- Ferrocerium rods
- Magnifying glass
- Ax

- Charring tins
- Fire starters (cotton, cardboard, lint from the dryer, etc.)

Tools for Food

Tools for food will include tools for hunting, cleaning, cooking, eating, and storing your food. The best tools are ones that allow you to accomplish many different tasks with that single tool, as this ensures you are not having to pack so many different things with you into the bush or around on hunting, trapping, or fishing trips.

- Knives
- Swiss Army Knife
- Whetstone
- Grinds
- Pots
- Skillet
- Meat rotisserie
- Planks
- Cast iron
- Cooking irons
- Stoves and burners
- Fishing wire
- Fish hooks
- Fishing rod (optional, a stick can be used if needed)

- Snare lines
- Bait
- Plates, bowls, and eating utensils
- Cooking utensils
- Stainless steel food storage containers
- Salt

Tools for Safety

Tools for safety include tools that will allow you to protect yourself in your camp, as well as tools that can be used in first aid situations. A well-stocked first-aid kit is important and should be in your G'n'G bag at all times.

- Bar soap
- Toothpaste
- Towels
- Bear spray
- Bear bangers
- First aid kit
    - 25 adhesive bandages in assorted sizes
    - 2 absorbent compress dressings (5 x 9 inches)
    - 2 triangular bandages
    - 1 adhesive cloth tape (10 yards x 1 inch)
    - 5 antiseptic wipes in individual packages

- 5 antibiotic ointment packets
- 2 packets of aspirin
- 2 hydrocortisone ointment packets
- 1 breathing barrier with a one-way valve
- 1 emergency blanket
- 1 instant cold compress
- 2 pairs of disposable gloves
- 1 3-inch gauze roll bandage
- 1 roller bandage, 4 inches wide
- 5 3 x 3-inch sterile gauze pads
- Oral thermometer (non-mercury and non-glass)
- Tweezers
- Emergency first aid guide
- Emergency radio

Tools for Travel

Tools for travel include all devices that will allow you to easily pack your materials into the bush. They also include all tools that will allow you to pack your materials through the forest, such as if you need to bring some things with you to forage, hunt, or fish for food.

- Bushcrafting backpack
- Bushcrafting vest (one for each person, properly sized)
- Canvas bags

- Smaller bags for organizing different things with (reusable shopping bags, small canvas bags, drawstring bags, etc.)

CHAPTER 5

The First Essential: Water

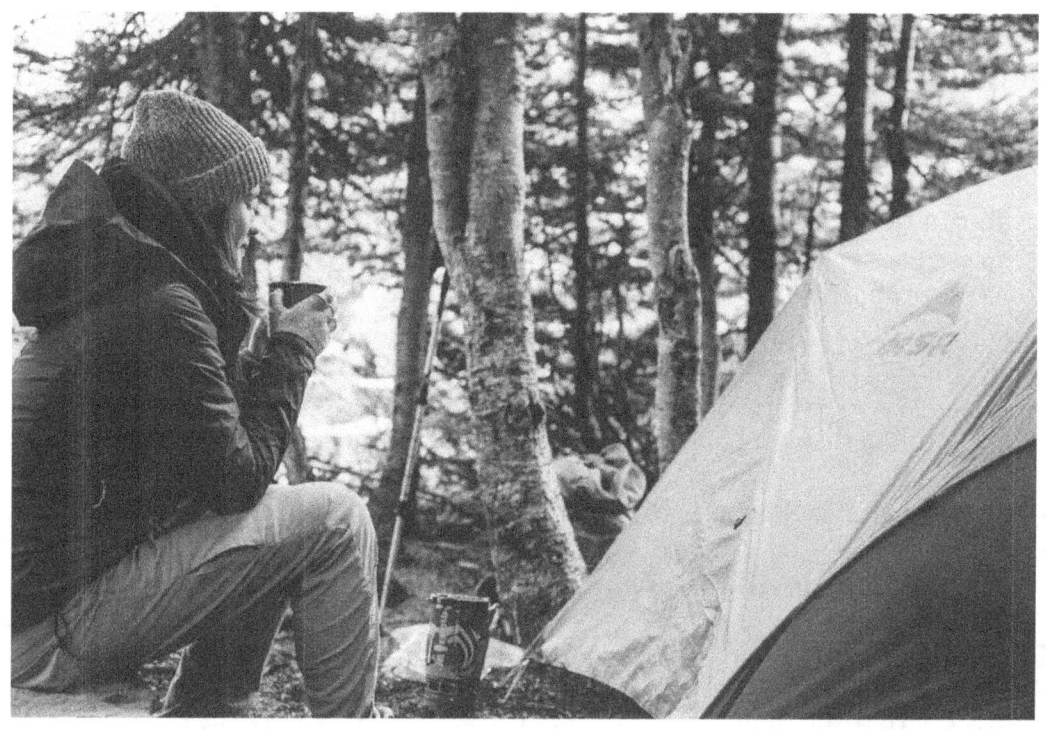

The very first thing you must have when escaping to the wilderness is to get there safely. We will discuss effective escaping methods in Chapter 10: The Great Escape. Once you have safely arrived at your survival location, you need to be able to access water. It is important that locating and accessing water is your first order of business, as this is going to enable you to find the perfect location to set your camp up in relation to the water. You always want to have your camp near water, even if you will only be there for a short period of time because it allows you to quickly and easily access the water itself. Water can be heavy, and hauling it back and forth from a water source to your camp can be exhausting and can expend energy that would be better used elsewhere.

Locating and Accessing Water

Hopefully, before you ever had to escape an urban situation, you had already surveyed a location for you to survive in, should the need arise. If not, however, it is relatively easy to source water in the bush. In the bush, you will be looking for a river, stream, or waterfall as these are all rapid-moving bodies of water that are likely to have fewer diseases and parasites in them. Lakes, ponds, marshes, and puddles should all be very last resorts, as they are likely full of disease and parasites since they cannot be filtered as easily as moving bodies of water can be. You can also catch rainwater in a container if you are in an area where rainfall is abundant. If you are in a dire situation, you can also look for an area that has fairly moist ground, and then you can try digging until you find water, however, there is no guarantee that this will work and it will expend a large amount of energy. As well, just because water is moving does not mean it is clean and safe for you to drink. You will need to purify your water with purifying drops, a purifying filter, or at the very least, by boiling it for 10 minutes before consuming it. Even moving water can be contaminated, and contamination can lead to illness or even death in unfortunate circumstances.

To source a moving body of water, take a look at the landscape around you. Particularly dry plants suggest that you are in an area where water is further away. If you can spot vegetation that is known for growing closer to water, such as mint, cattails, or ferns, you are likely close to a body of water. In this case, follow this patch of plants until you locate the water that they are growing around. Another great way to find water is to look for animal trails. Animals require water to survive. Well-worn paths in the forest indicate that you have located an "animal highway," or popular animal trail. Follow these trails to locate a water source. Look at the foliage to ensure that you are walking toward the water and not away from it.

If you do not rapidly come across a body of water, the next best thing to do is stop searching for water and start searching for altitude. Start walking up the highest piece of landscape you see, that you can reasonably walk up. Once you are well above the lower terrain, you will be able to look out across the land and get your bearings. You should be able to see water from this point, either through the body of water itself, or the clear distinction of well-hydrated vegetation. Again, it should be quite obvious as it will appear well-hydrated and deep green in color. Once you spot water, pinpoint landmarks, so you know exactly which direction to walk in order to get to the water. When you begin walking, ensure that you follow these milestones exactly, so you do not find yourself lost.

If you are still unable to source water, the next thing you must do is track animals. Be slow and steady, as animals will flee if they think they are being tracked, as they will believe you are hunting them. Taking your time and following the animals carefully will almost always lead you to a body of water, as animals will visit water several times per day to stay hydrated, since animals require hydration, too. While tracking animals, be very aware of your surroundings as remaining too focused on the animals you are tracking could leave you vulnerable to exposure, either with dangerous landscape features or with other animals who may be simultaneously tracking you.

Purifying and Storing Water

Properly purifying your water and storing it is essential. Failure to purify your water can lead to you consuming contaminated water and falling ill or being infected with parasites. Failing to store your water safely can lead to new contaminants being introduced to your water, which can also result in you falling ill. For short term survival situations, a large stainless steel water bottle or canteen is plenty for storing your water with. You should have one container per person, but containers can be shared if you were unable to bring more with you. You will simply need to refill the container more frequently to ensure everyone has access to adequate water.

Purifying your water can be done four different ways in the bush. Filtered bottles or purifying drops or tablets are the most common short term water purifying solutions in the bush, as they will instantly purify your water and protect you from contaminants. Both of these items can be purchased from a camping supply store or a military supply store, and they can be safely stored within your G'n'G gear for extended periods.

If you do not have access to purifying devices, there are two additional methods you can use for purifying your water in the bush. The preferred method is by fashioning a filter using materials from nature, while the latter is used in any purifying circumstance but can work on its own in a pinch. To create your own filter, take a cotton t-shirt and lay it over the top of a stainless steel pot. Then, you will take charcoal out of the bottom of your campfire and make a generous layer over the cotton shirt. If you can, have someone holding the shirt taut, so it covers the top of the pot, without falling in or having your filter tools fall off. Next, you will layer small gravel, dirt, and finally grass over the shirt. Then, you will pour water through this shirt, and it will land into the pot below. While you could technically drink this water now, it is possible that it is still contaminated, so it is best to boil the water afterward. Which, by the way, is the last option for purifying your water. Boiling your water on a heavy-rolling boil for at least 10 minutes ensures that it is safe enough for your consumption. Do not boil it for any less than that, and ensure that it remains on a full rolling boil so that you safely kill off any bacteria or parasites that may be contaminating your water. If you were unable to store your water in an airtight container, you will need to do this anytime you are about to drink it as new parasites or bacteria could be introduced to improperly stored water.

The proper storage solution for purified water is an airtight stainless steel bottle or canteen, as these will keep your water safe for drinking. You may need to purify water frequently if you only have small storage bottles, though you can always store larger amounts close to camp, so you do not have to haul water back so frequently. This way, while you still have to boil the water consistently, you are not wasting energy going back and forth to the water source several times per day or week.

Building Your Camp Near a Body of Water

Once you have located a water source, you need to decide where you will set up camp. It is important to concern yourself with this factor before doing much else, as this will help you decide where you will set up your fire and get yourself situated so that you can purify your water. Your camp should always be above the water line, and away from water runoffs enough that the ground will not be wet where you are camping. A wet ground can rapidly lead to illness, as it keeps you wet and damp for long periods of time, which is dangerous for your health. Your feet and face, especially, need to be kept dry. Excessive moisture around your face or feet can lead to infections. In the facial area, you run the risk of respiratory infection, whereas, around the feet, you run the risk of gangrene. Both can be fatal.

You also need to keep your camp away from the most common wildlife corridor. Bodies of water will always attract wildlife, and if you are not careful, you may place yourself on active trails, which can lead to you getting far too many wild visitors to your camp. While wildlife is unavoidable in the wilderness, you can situate yourself away from the main trails and corridors to ensure you are not directly in a busy place for wildlife to visit. You can tell if an area is busy for wildlife because you will notice a large amount of scat, fur, scratch marks, broken branches, and other signs that this is a place that is frequented by many critters.

If you build your camp uphill from a body of water, build your camp far enough back that if a landslide happened, you would not fall into the water or be crushed in the process. Soil erosion can lead to water banks being rather finicky, and if you are too close to a water bank, the weight of you walking along that space can result in the bank giving out and you falling in. This could lead to many dangers, ranging from hypothermia to drowning, or other water-related illnesses, injuries, or deaths.

Lastly, you need to consider how your water is going to be accessed and brought back to your camp. Based on where you have situated yourself, is it easy for you to take a large pot or basin down to the water source and bring it back to camp? You can guarantee this by looking for a trail that is easy to access and following that trail down to the water. Then, you need to consider how capable you will be of bringing the water back to camp, and how safe it will be for you to do so. Be careful about wildlife and soil erosion when collecting water, too, as something as simple as walking up an eroding bank or past unexpecting wildlife can lead to injuries or fatalities. If it is reasonable for you to access the water, the water does not pose a threat, and you have considered all other circumstances, you have found the perfect location for building your camp.

Securing Long-Term Access to Water

For long-term survival, you need to set up long-term access to water. This means you need to have a large, steady supply of water coming in that can be purified in large batches and stored safely so that it can be consumed. There are several ways that you can ensure safe access to drinking water, though many of these ways will require you to have proper storage containers for you to use in these situations. We will discuss options for if you have an abundance of tools or resources at your disposal, as well as options for if you don't so that you know how you can safely store water for long periods of time.

If you have an abundance of resources on hand, you can store water rather easily. Carrying larger containers of water from your water source back to camp, purifying them, and storing them in stainless steel, aluminum, high-density polyethylene (HDPE) containers, or uncracked glass containers enables you to store large amounts of water at once. This way, you can fetch, purify, and store water a few times a week rather than a few times a day, which saves plenty of time, energy, and resources.

If the area you are staying in experiences high amounts of rainfall, you can also collect rainwater for purifying. Rainwater tends to be cleaner than other water sources because it came straight from the sky and never had the chance to settle and become contaminated with things on the ground, or animals who may have interacted with it once it reached the ground. With that being said, you will need a rather large container to reasonably capture rainwater in, or at least several smaller containers that are capturing rainwater. You will also need to have access to a spot that is not covered by trees or brush so that the containers are directly exposed to the sky. If your water is falling through the trees first, it may become contaminated by bird feces, animals who are living in the trees, or other contaminants that could find their way into your water source. When it is not actively raining, you should cover your rain barrels to prevent contamination from vegetation, bugs, and animals.

If you do not have containers that you can store water in for extended periods of time, the next best thing you can do is set up a system for purifying your water each morning. Keep your homemade charcoal filter readily available next to a pot near your stove or the fire, as well as extra charcoal from the fire available for filtration. Then, each morning, your first order of business should be to collect water for the day. Go early enough that it is not too hot, but not so early that you encounter all of the wildlife accessing their first morning drink, which will likely happen around dawn and for an hour or two after. Once you have gathered your water, bring it back, filter it, and consume your water. Each evening, keep one or two containers filled with enough water for everyone and sterilize the other ones in boiling water. Rotate which ones are being sterilized in the evening to ensure they are both receiving adequate cleanings between usages.

It may take more work to access and store your water this way, but water is a non-negotiable when it comes to survival. Working into an efficient system ensures that you have access to all of the water you need, without having to expend any added energy getting it. This also ensures that you never miss a step and that you never go without.

In long-term survival situations, if you have purifying drops or tablets on hand, they should be preserved for dire circumstances, rather than used at camp. At camp, use a homemade charcoal filter and boiling method for purifying your water in large quantities. The filter or purifying drops and tablets can be preserved for days when you may need to venture away from camp, such as for fishing or hunting. This way, you do not have to transport an excess of fire starting materials and pots around with you to purify your water on the go.

CHAPTER 6

The Second Essential: Shelter

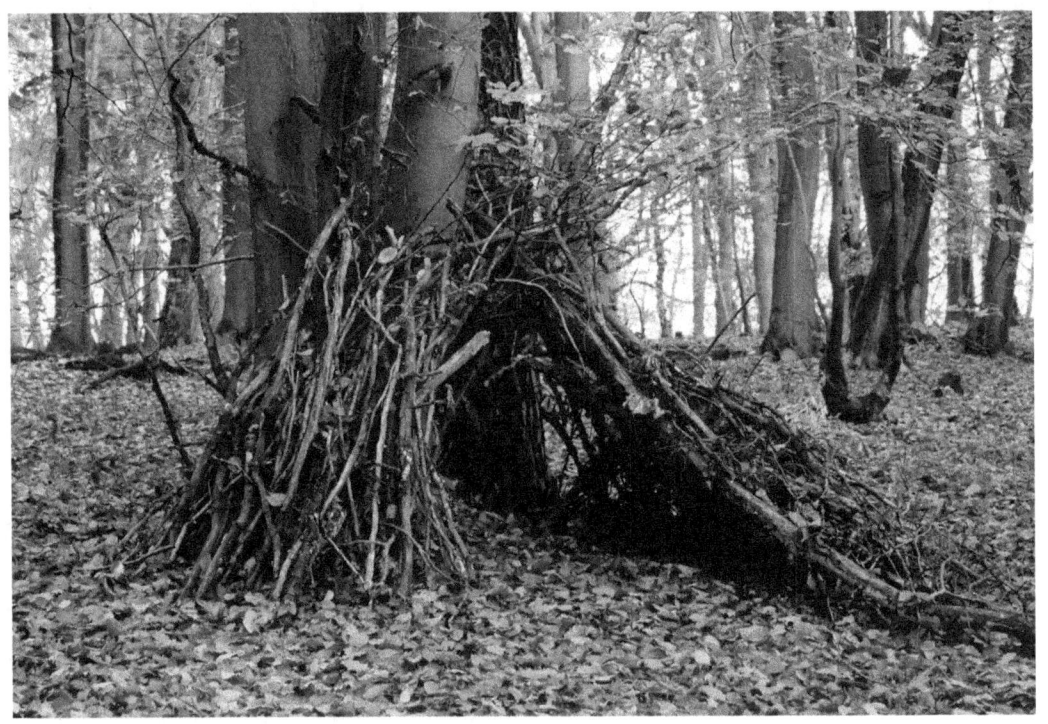

As soon as you have secured water, you need to secure a place to build your shelter, too. Your shelter, as you know, should be relatively close to a body of water, but not so close that it becomes hazardous. Aside from that, there are many other things to consider when it comes to building your shelter. Hardy individuals will advise that your shelter is merely a place to lay your head at night and that you should not think too much about it. I don't believe this is adequate advice, as it ignores the notion that our shelters are often our homes, and our homes provide a great sense of comfort and relief when they are built appropriately. In a normal, everyday situation, your home is where you live, and it provides you with a sense of comfort and security to live there, which is why you are able to unwind and tend to your mental and emotional needs. In the wilderness, your shelter will serve as your home for as long as you need it to, and you require it to offer the same mental and emotional solace. Being able to nurture your own mind and emotions in a survival situation is imperative, as it prevents you from running yourself into total burnout and then failing to have the energy required to get through the situation at hand.

Aside from the fact that your shelter should be properly built and designed in such a way that provides security, comfort, and relief, there are many other things that need to be factored into the building process. How much effort you put into it and what you do to build your shelter will depend on how long you will be surviving there for, and what materials you have available for you. If you were able to escape with a well-packed G'n'G bag, you should have plenty of tools you can rely on to help set up your camp. These tarps, ground covers, ropes and cordages, axes, and other materials will make building your shelter far easier. If you did not escape with your G'n'G bag, or if tools are missing out of it, you can make an adequate shelter out of everything in the bush, so there is no need to worry if you had to escape and were unable to bring your tools with you, or if you later realized your tools were inadequate or damaged.

Where to Build Your Shelter

The first thing you must be aware of when it comes to building your shelter is knowing where to build it. You already know how to situate your shelter near a body of water, but there are many other things to consider, too. The wilderness can pose many dangers that you need to consider if you are going to be able to safely survive for any period. Build shelter away from immediate dangers, as well as less-obvious dangers, to avoid harming anyone at your camp. Improperly located shelters can and do, lead to serious injuries and even fatalities. It may sound excessive if you have never been in the wilderness, but it is a reality, and unfortunately, it hurts and injures thousands every year. Anything from falling trees to wildlife and other dangers can present themselves and result in fatalities in the bush, which is directly contradictory to your desire to survive.

Finding the best place to set up your camp requires you to know about widowmakers or dangers that can instantly kill anyone in your camp, including yourself. In the bush, the most common widowmaker is a tree or tree branch that has begun falling down but has yet to fall all the way down. Dead trees also pose a danger, as they are weak and can easily be blown over or broken in various weather conditions, which can lead to them falling. If you were to build your shelter under or even near this tree or tree branch, it could fall at any time and instantly injure or kill anyone who was under it. It is imperative that you look around at the trees surrounding you when you are building your shelter, and when you are moving around the wilderness in general, so you can steer clear of potential hazards such as falling trees or tree branches. As well, never underestimate the weight and power behind a tree branch. Even a seemingly small branch can deliver a massive blow, especially if it falls quite a ways, which can lead to injury or sudden death.

Landslides, rockslides, and other slides can also lead to instant injury or death in the bush. If you camp somewhere and there is a sheer rock face, a large rocky mountain, or any other rock formation nearby, you are at risk of that rock formation coming down and burying you, and anyone you are with, under the rocks. Those would also result in instant death. If you were at the top of a terrain that began to slide, you could drop to your death, be struck by something on your way down, or land in water and drown.

You should also beware of wildlife and insects. Wildlife can attack you when you are not paying attention, which can lead to instant death, and certain insects or ground critters can bite you, which can lead to deadly infections. Black widows or brown recluse spiders, for example, can bite, which can lead to your skin dying off, which ultimately turns into a disease that will kill you within hours or days, at best. If you can, keep your bed up and away from the ground, and inspect it before ever getting into it to avoid having any insects or small animals getting into your bedding and harming you. You should also keep the bedding tightly tucked in around you to avoid loose bedding, welcoming dangerous insects into your space.

The best place for your shelter is on dry, flat ground that is naturally sheltered by healthy trees that show no signs of decay or falling down. You can clean away the underbrush from the area to ensure the ground is clear and easy to walk and build on, and less likely to attract bugs and small animals since they prefer dead leaves and other vegetation to hide under. Stay away from large boulders, rock formations, or bodies of water as they can pose a threat to your camp. As well, stay away from common wildlife corridors, marked by frequently used trails, as being too close could result in you attracting dangerous wildlife to your camp.

Short Term Shelter Solutions

If you are surviving for a short period of time, a simple tarp tent with a ground cloth should be plenty to protect you for as long as you need. There are three tarp tents you can make with a tarp, rope, and some rocks or sticks that will help you stake the tarp to the ground. They are easy to make, provide adequate shelter, and are excellent for short term survival situation, including short term overall survival or short term hunting or fishing trips away from your long-term camp. The three tarp tents you can make include a tarp lean-to, a supported flying tarp, or a low lying flying tarp. Each of these shelters can be used for different purposes, and they are all simple to make.

A tarp lean-to can be made by locating four trees that are relatively close together, and that form a square between them. To create your lean-to, you will simply tie each corner of the tarp to the tree, pulling it tight, so it forms a nice taut surface. One half of the tarp should be tied at least one foot higher than the other half. This protects you from rain, as anything that falls on the slanted tarp will immediately fall off rather than leaking, or adding weight to the tarp and eventually causing it to cave in. If you are in an area with any breeze, build the shorter side of the lean-to toward the breeze, so it keeps you protected from the elements.

A supported flying tarp can be made by locating the middle of one of the sides of your tarp and tying it about four to five feet up the trunk of a medium-sized tree. You will then take either corner from the same side that has been tied to the tree and pull it out to a 45-degree angle from the tree and keep it in place using medium to large rocks on the edges of the tarp. The side of the tarp that is opposite the tree should be weighed down by rocks, too. You can tuck the tarp underneath itself and weigh it down with rocks from the inside, as this can prevent precipitation from getting into your shelter.

A low lying flying tarp is made the same way as a supported flying tarp, except that it is far lower to the ground. For a low lying flying tarp, you will tie it only two to three feet up the tree trunk, and you will keep the openings on either side fairly small by folding the corners of the tarp underneath itself and weighing it down from the inside using rocks. You will continue to fold the opposite edge under and weigh it down with rocks, too. This smaller tarp allows for one or two people to sleep snug, prevents wind from being able to get into the tarp, and makes it far less likely that any predators will try to get into your tent and bother you while you are sleeping.

No matter how you position your tarp, you should always clean away the ground underneath the tarp and lay a ground cloth under it. Thick canvas, animal hide, woolen blankets, or other coverings will prevent the cold or damp ground from affecting you while you sleep. You should place these ground cloths even if you have access to a sleeping bag, as they ensure that you are able to stay as warm and protected from the elements as possible.

Long-Term Shelter Solutions

If you are going to need to survive long term, or if you do not have access to a tarp or ground cloths, there are many ways that you can build a shelter out of the resources offered from the land. Branches, leaves, brush, dirt and clay, rocks, and other materials can all be used to form excellent shelters that keep you protected from the elements and offer comfort and security in the wilderness. One excellent element of these shelters, too, is that they are structured out of natural materials, which means that you are better camouflaged into the environment. This way, you are less likely to grab the interest of nearby wildlife and are more likely to remain hidden and left alone when you are in your shelter.

Building a shelter from resources in the forest will vary depending on what you have access to, how big of a shelter you need, and where you are. Rather than attempting to give you specific step-by-step instructions to build various shelters, I will explain how you can improvise and build your own walls, roof, and floor using resources you find in the bush. This way, you know how to improvise and make your own shelter in your own terrain.

Before you build anything for your shelter, clean the ground around where the shelter will be placed. Remove leaves, branches, rocks, and any debris that will interrupt the ground space, as all of this will be too messy for the floor of your shelter. You will want soft, clear space that is less likely to harbor insects or sharp sticks or rocks that could cut your skin or cause bruises or other injuries. In the bush, even minor injuries can become major problems, so you need to avoid them at all costs.

Begin building your shelter with the walls by creating walls that are strong and resistant enough to keep wind and other elements out of your shelter. You will want to build your walls based on the elements you are likely to be exposed to, as minor windy conditions will require much less protection than heavy rainfall or snow. Build your walls based on the worst elements you are most likely to be exposed to so they are adequate for every situation. They also need to be strong enough to hold up the roof you create for your shelter. Your walls should be four-sided like a conventional house. However, there is one type of shelter where they can be adapted, and where they should actually be put on second instead of first. That is, you would build an A-frame roof and build the walls up on the front and back of it. These are great shelters for areas where there is high precipitation or where it is cold, so you want to have a small shelter that does not have a lot of room for wind or other elements to get in. These can also be useful if you are in an area that lacks natural resources such as trees and brush, as they do not require as many materials.

As you build up the walls of your shelter, use larger branches to make the main walls themselves. You can plant the ends in the ground, so they stand up, and then use a rope to tie the branches together if you have any. Then, you can weave small leafy branches, twigs, or pine-covered branches into the larger branches to create insulation and to protect your shelter from the elements. If you have any, extra tarps or ground cloths can also be used to cover the walls; however, the majority of your tarps and ground cloths, if you have them, should be reserved for the roof and floor as these are more important uses for those materials. If you do not have branches to build your walls with, you can build them out of dirt, clay, or snow. Ensure that any shelters made out of these materials are made with thick walls and that they are made in a way where they are unlikely to collapse. Packing down the building materials and giving dirt or clay plenty of time to dry out ensures that they are less likely to collapse.

For your roof, you want to use small to medium branches, and as few as possible. Medium or larger branches could fall through if too much weight were to come on them or if your structure were to be weak somewhere, and those branches could then cause serious injuries. It is better to use long, small to medium branches sparingly to make a basic frame for your roof. Then, you can cover the roof in leafy branches, evergreen branches, grass, large leaves, or anything else you can find that will create a nice thick cover. Be sure to use a few layers of your roof materials to build your roof, as this ensures that precipitation and weather elements cannot penetrate your roof and cause you to get wet inside. As well, ensure you do not let the roof get too heavy as this will lead to it collapsing and possibly causing an injury. Always make your roof in an A-frame shape, or in a lean-to shape with one side shorter than the other, as this will allow precipitation to naturally fall off and will prevent any damaged parts of your roof from falling directly on you. If you have a spare tarp, you can use, place a tarp over the roof frame but under the natural materials, as this will provide an added layer of protection from the weather, without attracting attention to your shelter.

Lastly, you need to build the floor. The floor should be built at the end because this way, you can quickly go through and sweep out any building materials that may have fallen into your floor when you were building your shelter. Once you have cleaned out the floor of your shelter, you need to insulate it, too. In the wilderness, the ground holds a lot of moisture, even if you have built a shelter over it. Covering the ground with dry materials ensures that you are not exposed to that moisture. In addition to moisture, the ground can become quite cold, which can lead to your body temperature dropping. Proper insulation in your shelter can prevent this. The best materials to use to insulate your floor are soft brush, such as small branches covered in leaves or evergreen branches. Shake them out to eliminate bugs, and then lay your ground cloth over them if you have one to keep yourself insulated. If you are going to be surviving for extended periods of time, you can also dry and cure any pelts you get from animals you trap or hunt, and then layer those pelts over the floor of your shelter. Excess can also be layered over the walls and on the ceiling of your shelter, as the more you have, the warmer your shelter will be. Again, be cautious not to place too much on your roof or hang too much from your ceiling, as this can cause it to collapse, and that could cause injury or worse.

CHAPTER 7

The Third Essential: Fire

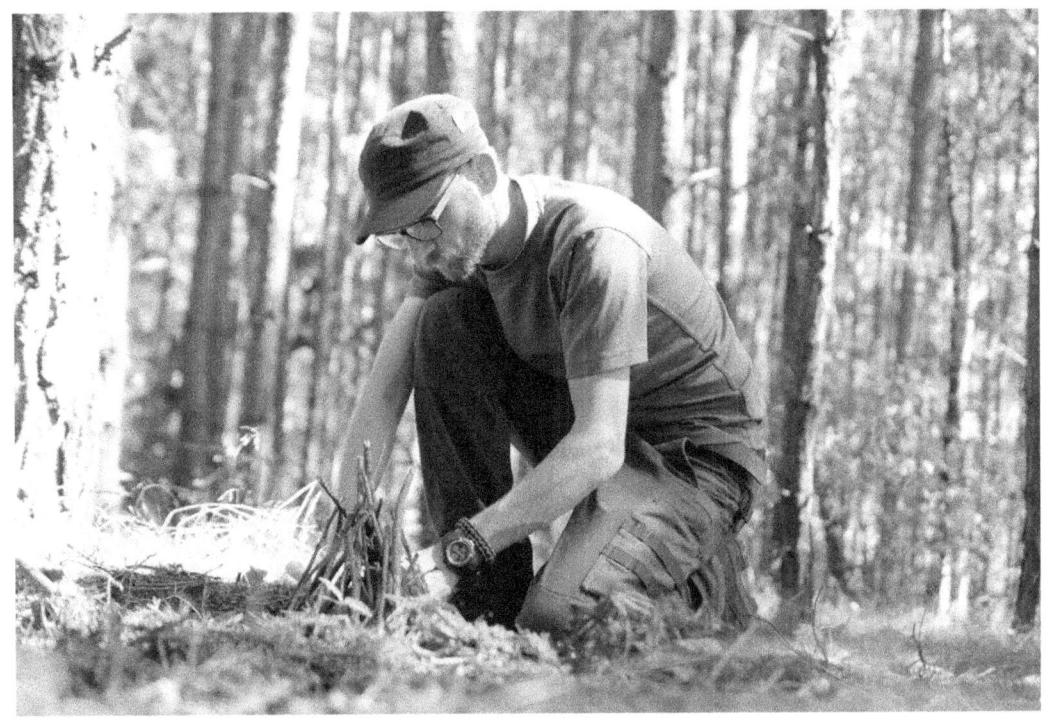

After you have your water and shelter figured out, you need fire. Fire is an essential element to survival as it allows you to maintain a proper core body temperature, allows you to cook your foods to safe eating temperatures, and provides you with the opportunity to sterilize things. In the wilderness, smoke baths are a great way to cleanse yourself and sterilize yourself of any bacteria, as smoke is known for creating an acidic environment and eliminating harsh bacteria. Fire provides an abundance of benefits in the bush, so long as you have built the right fire for the purpose you require because, like anything, fire is a tool for survival.

For short term survival situations, you should be able to use your fire-starting materials that you brought with you. Your lighter is good to start your fire, and you can forage for wood in the forest around so that you have fuel for it. Brush like leaves, evergreen branches, and even some brambles are excellent for keeping small fires going for short survival experiences.

If you are in a long-term survival situation, you will need to have more supplies on hand to help you with your fire. Building up a stock of cut wood and giving it time to dry out, and keeping plenty of kindling and fire starter on hand will be important. You should also know how to use a magnifying glass to start a fire, as well as have a ferrocerium rod, or a flint rod, which can start fires without the need for matches or lighters. This way, you have everything you need to start as many fires as are required.

Where to Build Your Fire

There are a few different areas where you will build a fire during a survival situation. In short term survival situations, building a fire directly in your camp, about three feet away from your shelter, is plenty to keep you warm and dry. A fire should be built in this same location if you are staying long-term. However, this will be the only fire that you will need in a short term situation. Any situation that will last longer than 24 hours, or where you will need to actually cook over your open fire, will require you to have a fire built elsewhere, too.

Food fires should always be built at least 100 yards away from your shelter, so that as you cook your food, you are not attracting predators to your actual camp. Understand that even after the fire is out and everything has been cleaned, the smell of cooked food will linger on everything that was around or has come into contact with that fire or any tools used to cook food over or around that fire. In fact, this is why you should also have separate clothes that you use for cooking, and they should be stored away from your shelter, too.

Another place where you may want to build a fire would be if you were away from camp hunting or fishing and needed to build a fire for warmth, water purification, or cooking food on the go. These fires are usually much smaller, require fewer materials, so they are easier to start and maintain. Aside from these three areas, you should not require any further fires in your survival experience.

Building a Birds Nest

The first step for building any fire is to have adequate fire-starting materials. Many fire starter materials can be collected from home, while others can be gathered from the bush. In the bush, things like pine needles, dry moss, and dry grass or brush can be used to start a fire.

From home, the fire starter materials you can bring include:

- Crumpled or shredded paper
- Cotton balls
- Tampons
- Cotton, linen, and other plant-based material
- Dryer lint
- Wood shavings
- Greasy chips
- Cardboard
- Pinecones
- Wax from candles

A great way to create fire starters is to take a cardboard toilet paper roll and cut it into 3 sections. Then, fill the center of the toilet paper roll with dryer lint, cotton balls, or scraps of plant-based materials. Cover the entire thing in candle wax to keep it all sealed together and then store it in a plastic bag so it does not get wet. You can make as many of these as possible and bring them all with you for starting your fires with.

If you do not have fire-starting materials from home, the bush has plenty to offer. The most common way to make a fire starter in the wilderness is to make what survivalists call a "birds nest." Birds' nests are made in pretty much the same way a bird would actually make their nest. You will take twigs and scraps of vegetation off of the ground and weave it together into a bird's nest shape. The shape allows for plenty of oxygen to move through the starting materials, while also keeping them close enough together that the fire can reasonably spread through the materials.

Once you have made the bird's nest, it will be placed in your fire so you can start the fire itself. Despite the fact that the bird's nest is responsible for starting the fire, it should be the last thing you place in your fire as you want to keep it safe from being damaged in case one of your fire logs falls on it. Instead, you will start by clearing space on the ground for you to place your fire, and then you will surround the fire with rocks so that it does not travel and cause a major fire in the bush. Next, you will build your log formation in the fire pit. Then, you will place the bird's nest in the log formation and start that on fire. This will then catch fire and eventually catch your logs on fire, giving you a steady, strong fire that can be maintained for long periods of time.

Just like with the initial log formation, the starter and log formation themselves do not need to be maintained after the fire is started. It is perfectly fine that the bird's nest completely burns away and that the logs fall out of formation as they burn away. Simply place new logs over the fire in a way that prevents them from smothering the fire, so plenty of oxygen can get in and help the fire spread to the new logs. This way, your fire can last for as long as you need it to.

Fire for Heat

Fire that is created for keeping you warm needs to be made in a way where you can easily sit around it, and where you can trust that it will be long-lasting. If you are trying to keep warm outside of your shelter, you want your fire to be no more than three feet tall, but no less than about one and a half feet tall. Any taller than three feet and your fire runs the risk of catching the forest itself on fire, while anything smaller than one and a half feet can run the risk of it burning out and leading to you getting cold. Overnight, you want a proper fire that can last for hours without going out so that as you sleep, you can stay warm. The only time this may not be true is if you are surviving in an area where the temperatures do not drop any lower than about 15 degrees, as you can use your sleeping bag to keep you warm and comfortable during the night. Anything lower, though, and you will need a long-lasting fire for heat.

For daytime, the best fire lays for heat include the teepee fire lay, the lean-to fire lay, or the log cabin fire lay. The long-burning fire lay and the Dakota fire pit are also excellent for keeping you warm, with the long-burning fire working overnight, and the Dakota fire pit keeping you warm during windy conditions.

Teepee Fire Lay

The teepee fire lay is the most common fire lay that people think of. It is frequently taught in scouts and other survival programs, and it offers excellent fire for warmth. This fire lay is not good for cooking because it is too tall, it gets too hot, and it does not offer a reliable location for cooking your food over.

To build the teepee fire lay, prepare your fire location by clearing the ground and outlining the fire pit with rocks. Then, start by taking kindling-size branches that are about 1 foot long each and build a teepee shape with them, crossing them at the top ends to keep them in place. If you can, find a piece of kindling with a "Y" shape at the end and use that as your starting point. Make sure you keep the kindling far enough apart that plenty of oxygen can get through.

Once you have built a teepee out of kindling, you will need to build a teepee out of branches, or fuel logs. Again, keep these branches far enough apart that oxygen can get through easily, as oxygen is essential to your fire being able to start and thrive.

Finally, place your bird's nest in the center of the kindling teepee and light it on fire. It will burn, catch the kindling on fire, and then the kindling will catch your fuel logs on fire. Add fresh fuel logs one at a time to keep the fire going, and add them carefully to avoid smothering the fire you have already started.

Lean-to Fire Lay

A lean-to fire lay is an excellent fire lay that is easy to build, that offers plenty of oxygen for your fire to grow, and that makes it extremely easy for you to get your starter in the bottom of your fire lay. To build a lean-to fire, you need to clear your space for your fire to be placed, then you need to place one larger log on an angle, propped up against kindling or a small rock. Next, you will layer larger kindling or small fuel logs over that leaning branch. You will lean the ends up around them, creating a half-circle of logs in such a way that they look like a small shelter or a lean-to. Your lean-to should get shorter and smaller on the end near the ground, and longer or taller on the end at the top of the propped-up stick.

Once you have set up your lean-to fire lay, you can place your bird's nest in the opening made from the propped up log. Then, you will light the bird's nest on fire. It will catch your kindling pieces on fire, and then the larger fuel log that is holding the fire lay in place. As you place logs over the fire, be careful not to smother them.

Log Cabin Fire Lay

A log cabin fire lay is a simple crisscross style fire lay that has a teepee shape built inside of it. Your log cabin fire lay is not particularly tall, but it does offer plenty of fuel to keep it going for long periods of time. A well-built log cabin fire lay should last several hours, at least. While it is not enough for an overnight fire, it will get you plenty of warmth.

To create a log cabin fire lay, you will start by sourcing several pieces of kindling, and then approximately 10 pieces of fuel logs that are about one and a half to two feet long. You will first make a teepee shape with kindling in the center of your cleaned fire pit that has been sectioned off with larger rocks. Then, you will lay two of your fuel logs beside your fire, on opposite sides, running lengthwise across the fire pit. Next, you will stack two of your fuel fire logs across the edges of the two you originally laid, creating a square-shape with the logs now. Lay two logs over the same direction as your original two logs, then two crisscross over those. Lay two more logs in the same direction as your original two logs. You should have 10 logs in a log cabin shape around your teepee, and a well-built teepee in the middle.

Now, all you need to do is place your bird's nest in the center of the teepee and light it on fire. The fire will catch the kindling, then eventually, the kindling will catch the log cabin shape, and it will start to burn. Because of the formation, it should last several hours if you used large enough fuel logs.

Long Burning Fire Lay

A long burning fire lay is excellent for keeping you warm all night long. It is achieved by digging out a long pit, filling it with fuel logs, and burning it from one end to the other. The idea is that you start a slow fire with a controlled amount of oxygen, and the result is the fire burns all night long. To create a long burning fire lay for yourself, you will start by digging a narrow ditch about 6 feet long. It should be wide enough to hold logs, and long enough that it runs at least the length of your body.

Once you have dug the ditch, you want to source fuel logs that can be placed along the ditch itself. Make sure they reach from one end to the other, so you have a six foot length of logs that will be burnt overnight. Leave about a foot of space at the end of the ditch without any fuel logs, and create a teepee fire lay in that space using smaller kindling, and then larger kindling. Then, place your bird's nest in the teepee formation and light it on fire. As it burns, ensure that the edge of your first fuel log is placed close enough that it catches on fire from your kindling fire. Once it catches, you can trust that the entire six foot log fire will burn throughout the night, keeping you warm while you sleep.

Dakota Fire Pit

Dakota fire pits are excellent for inconspicuous fires, or fires built in windy areas. The way the pit is built, the fire remains relatively unseen and unaffected by elements like wind. These firepits are also excellent for cooking over, as you can make the surface area of the fire rather small, and it is level with the ground, which means you can place a pan over it and allow it to cook using the heat from your fire.

To create a Dakota fire pit, you will start by sourcing small pieces of kindling. You want a large amount, as it is unlikely that you will be creating a large fire pit for your fire. If you were to create your fire pit too large, it would defeat the purpose, and the wind would still pose a threat to your fire. Instead, you want to dig a pit about 1 foot across and 1.5 feet deep. Then, you will move about 2 feet away from the pit you have dug and dig another pit at an angle, aiming toward the bottom of your original pit. Once you are about to connect the two, use your hand to dig away any dirt that remains between your two pits so you can connect them without collapsing the dirt above your newly formed tunnel. It is important that your tunnel is at least as thick as your arm, if not a little larger, as this is where your fire will receive the oxygen it needs to thrive. Without this oxygen tunnel, your fire pit would lack oxygen, and your fire would burn out.

Once your pit and tunnel are properly built, you can go ahead and build a teepee fire shape in the main pit. Add your bird's nest into the bottom of the teepee and light it on fire. If you need to, you can reach your arm through the oxygen tunnel and light the bird's nest on fire this way to avoid burning yourself. You can continue adding smaller pieces of wood into your pit as needed, as the oxygen tunnel will continue to fuel your fire with enough oxygen each time you add a new log. Simply make sure you do not add such a thick log that the entire main pit is filled, as you will still fail to get enough oxygen into your fire if you do this.

Fire for Cooking

The Dakota fire pit is an excellent all-around fire for warmth and cooking. There are two additional fire lays you can use, however, which will also help you with cooking food at your camp. Note that while you could technically cook over any fire, safely placing your cookware over the fires would be challenging, and the size of the fires would result in your cookware becoming too hot and you instantly burning anything you attempted to cook. Cooking fires should be small and easy to contain, and they should burn hot yet slow, as you will not be cooking over the flame itself but rather over the embers at the bottom of the fire. This ensures that your food will be cooked all the way through without becoming burnt from the flames, and you will remain healthy.

Pyramid Fire Lay

The pyramid fire lay is similar to the log cabin one, except that instead of creating a teepee in the center and a log cabin around it, you will be using the same method of interlocking the logs and turning kindling-sized pieces of wood into a pyramid shape. To make your pyramid fire lay, look for several uniformed pieces of kindling that you can stack together to make your pyramid.

Once you have found your pieces, lay two pieces of kindling on the ground parallel to each other. Then, lay two parallel pieces in the opposite direction, over the edges of the original two pieces you laid down. Keep doing this, going back and forth in either direction, and moving the kindling closer and closer together until it comes together in the center, but leave a small gap open in the top. About halfway through, add a bird's nest into the bottom and make sure you leave gaps large enough that will let you catch the bird's nest starter on fire.

As soon as the fire lay is set up, you can light your bird's nest on fire and let the fire catch. The pyramid should burn down quickly, yet it is easy for you to keep it going as long as you need to in order to keep the embers hot. If the pyramid burns too low,

Star Fire With a Cooking Arm

A star fire with a cooking arm is a more advanced contraption, but it can still be made from the bush. To make your star fire with a cooking arm, you will start with the fire lay. The star fire lay requires you to have at least 4 fuel sized pieces of wood, though more is always better. You will bring one point from each piece of wood together in the center and evenly space the opposite points out around the center, making a star shape. Under the center of your star, you should dig out a small depression so that your fire has plenty of oxygen to keep it burning. You should also leave slight gaps between the ends of the logs, as this allows even more oxygen to flow through and keep your fire thriving.

In the center of your fire lay, you should keep the points separated by about a foot, so they create a circle but are not all touching in the very middle. Then, you will lay a bird's nest in the center and cover it loosely with some kindling.

Before you light your fire, you will want to find a large, sturdy Y-shaped branch and bury the single end down in the ground at least one foot. You can also stack rocks around it to prevent it from falling. You should place this stick about 2-3 feet away from your fire lay, facing toward the fire so that when you balance a branch between it, the branch points toward the center of your fire. The top of the Y-shape should be only about 3-4 feet high, as this will ensure that it is not too high for you to cook with. The branch itself should be thick enough that if you placed a loaded Dutch oven on it, it would not bend or break. Then, you want to find another large, but not too thick, branch that can be placed through the Y-shape, with one end up above the fire. If you can, bury the end of the single branch that will be hanging over the fire, or cover it with heavy rocks and other items that will prevent it from falling once you anchor a Dutch oven to the opposite end.

Now, start your fire by lighting the bird's nest and letting the kindling get going. Then, once it is going well, you can load up your Dutch oven or a steel pot and hang it on the branch itself. The fire should not be touching the bottom of the pot, but it should be high enough that the bottom of the pot is receiving consistent, high temperatures that will cook the contents inside of the pot. Be sure to use heavy duty cooking gloves or another branch to remove your pot from over the fire, as it will be extremely hot when you are done cooking with it.

CHAPTER 8

The Fourth Essential: Food

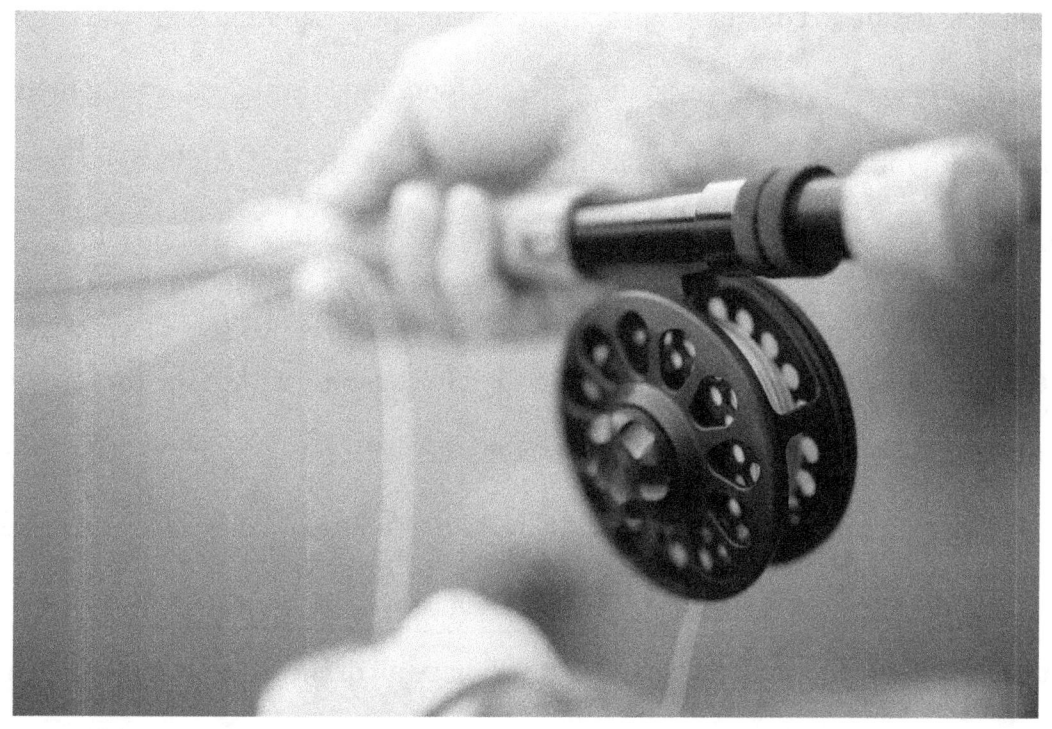

While you can last three weeks without food, the reality is that the energy it takes to survive in the bush is far greater than it takes to survive in an urban environment. Even if you are in an urban environment but have been cut off from your usual sources, you will find yourself burning a lot more energy to maintain your livelihood, which results in you burning more energy and needing more calories. Anytime you put excess demand on your body this way, it is essential to stock up on calories as quickly as possible to make up for the deficit. Otherwise, you could start seeing the negative symptoms of hunger caused by not eating. While it may take you three weeks to die of starvation, it only takes on average a few hours to start feeling the adverse side effects of not eating, and three to five days to start feeling wholly drained due to the lack of calories.

Eating in the bush can seem intimidating because you have to make sure that anything you are eating is safe to consume. Foraging for vegetation, catching fish, and trapping or hunting wildlife are all of the ways you will gain food, but if you do it wrong in any way, you could find yourself facing a nasty infection or parasite that could deteriorate your health, and fast. Fortunately, there are many steps you can take to ensure that eating in the bush will be safe and that you will remain healthy from the food you have consumed. As far as timelines go, you should aim to find food to consume within the first twenty-four hours of being on-site. If you need to, you can start with foraging for food as this is an excellent way to get the food you need quickly, and you do not have to rely on wildlife to take the bait and land in your trap or on your hook. Once you have done that, though, you need to start looking for animal protein as it will have all of the calories and nutrients that you need to keep your body going during those days where you are challenging your body more than usual.

Types of Food to Eat in the Wilderness

In the wilderness there are five types of food you can consume, four of which are considered an animal protein. The first type of food you can consume in the wilderness is foraged vegetation, including berries, herbs, vegetables, and other plants that are safe for human consumption. These are important as they provide you with an abundance of vitamins, which ensures that you have all of the vitamins and minerals that you need to thrive.

The four types of animal protein you can consume in the wilderness include fish, reptiles, birds, and small to medium mammals. While you could technically aim to hunt and destroy a more massive mammal unless you have adequate means for preserving that meat before it spoils, it is not generally a good idea. You could find yourself wasting the meat and attracting far too many predators to your camp.

Foraging for Vegetation

Foraging for vegetation is something that cannot be summarized in one single beginner's guide dedicated to survival as a whole. This particular topic contains so many nuances that are unique to your geographic area. The best way to safely forage for vegetation is to have a proper wildcrafting or foraging book that reflects your unique geographical region and to have that in your G'n'G bag so that you can bring it with you if you ever find yourself in a survivalist situation. If you want to be even safer, you can consider hiring a local herbalist or wildcrafter who is skilled with the local flora and who can show you what to look for and what to avoid. Nearly every plant has poisonous lookalikes that can lead to anything from minor illness or injury to severe illness or even death. It is imperative that you learn how to tell these plants apart, as this ensures you know how to safely forage from the forest without accidentally gathering something that could poison yourself and your entire camp. In short term survival situations, you may be able to survive without forage, but anything more than a few days should involve forage as you will need the extra vitamins and minerals from plants to avoid putting yourself at risk of malnutrition-related illness.

Once you have foraged, you will need to clean your vegetation for safe consumption and store it properly. Soak your harvest in already-filtered water for at least thirty minutes to eliminate unwanted bacteria and debris from it, then run the vegetation through additional filtered water so that you can remove anything off of the surface of your foraged goods. If you want to cook it into a meal, you can do that, too. Some vegetation is only safe to eat once it has been prepared, so be sure you are aware of the consumption rules around different flora before consuming it.

To store your vegetation, you want to use a breathable bag that you can seal to prevent insects or small animals from getting into your foraged food and consuming it or introducing unwanted bacteria to your harvested matter. While it is usually easy to access more vegetation, you do not want to expend any more energy than you need to, so if you are able to collect a fair amount of it at once, you will want to preserve it for a few days of eating.

One thing I do want to be sure you are aware of is the importance of ethical foraging. When foraging, even for a survival situation, it is imperative that you refrain from harvesting an entire crop of anything. Even if you believe there are many more crops in the forest, it is important that you never take more than about 10% of what is available. Over-harvesting can lead to those crops becoming depleted, and if you do find yourself in a long-term situation, it can lead to you not having enough to consume at later dates.

Further, even small instances of over-harvesting can disrupt the harmony of the forest and lead to long-term damage.

Hunting, Trapping, and Fishing

Hunting, trapping, and fishing are the three ways that you will get animal protein into your stomach in the woods. Trapping and fishing are usually the easiest, since hunting would require some form of weapon, and unless you already have weapons with you, it is challenging to make a homemade weapon strong enough to humanely kill a mammal without causing a large amount of suffering beforehand.

All trapping is accomplished using a snare, though the way the snare is set up will often differ depending on what you are trying to trap, and where you are setting the snare up. There are two important snare setups that you need to know about when it comes to trapping animals in the wilderness, which will ensure that you are successful in your endeavors. The first is a squirrel snare, and the second is a snare that will capture just about any other type of animal.

A squirrel snare is a series of traps created along a branch. To create one, you will start by finding a reasonably long branch that you can prop up against a tree, reaching to the lower branches of the tree you have propped your branch up on. Squirrels, by nature, will use this branch to get to the ground. Once you have your branch, you will take your snare line, twist a loop into one end of it, and feed the opposite end through your loop so that you have a slip knot. Then, you will fix the snare to the branch in a way that holds it open so that as the squirrel runs down the branch, they will be caught in the snare and effectively trapped. You should set multiple snares on a single branch to maximize your ability to catch squirrels.

A regular snare can be set by making another slip knot with your snare line. To do so, twist a loop into one end of your snare line and feed the opposite end through the loop, so you have a slip knot. Then, you need to look for animal highways or corridors. These usually look like well-worn paths that indicate that animals frequently use that particular area. Once you have found an animal highway or corridor, you want to follow a smaller worn-in trail that leads into the brush, as this indicates that it is routinely used by small to medium animals. Then, you want to fix the free line of your trap to a branch and set the snare so that it sits open over the path itself. This way, when a small mammal or bird runs down the trail, they will get caught in the snare line and die.

Anytime you set a snare, wear plastic over your hands, either using gloves or a garbage bag or wash your hands with dirt and charcoal to remove your scent. Humans do emit pheromones that animals can smell, and the second they pick up on your pheromones, they will stay far away from your snares, which will lead to failed trapping endeavors. If you do not have anything available, start a small fire about 50 yards away from your trapping site and let it burn long enough that you can harvest charcoal from it and use that. As it burns, stand directly in the smoke for a few minutes to help eliminate your scent from your clothes and the rest of your body, too.

If after a few days, your snares are not catching anything, you may need to adjust their location or set a piece of bait on the other side of the snare that will encourage an animal to reach through it. Be sure to use a form of bait that is nice and smelly, and that is made up of some sort of food item that is not easy to find in your area. For example, if you wanted to catch a small rodent, you might use sardine oil or something similar as a bait to encourage them to go through the trap. This way, the animal has more incentive, and your traps are more likely to catch a harvest.

Fishing is just as easy as trapping, if not easier. All you need to do is find a river, creek, or lake that has a nice deep pit in it where the water is not moving too quickly. Then, you want to tie a piece of fishing line around a branch that is around four to five feet long and two inches thick. Avoid thin branches, as they will snap under the weight of a fish.
When you have the right sized branch, tie a fishing line on one end with a hook on the end of it. Attach some bait to the hook, which can be anything from a small insect to a piece of raw game meat. Drop your baited line into the water and keep it slowly moving, so it behaves like live bait, which will encourage the fish to bite. It may take up to half an hour or even an hour to catch a fish, though if you wait any longer than that, it may mean that you are not in an optimal fishing location and need to search for somewhere better to catch your fish from.

Butchering Small to Medium Game

Once you have caught your animal, you need to know how to butcher it. Small to medium game is all butchered roughly the same, as their physical bodies are usually quite similar. For example, a rabbit, a rat, a squirrel, and a raccoon would all have similar body shapes and organ placements, meaning the butchering process would be more or less the same.

To butcher your small to medium game, you will start by hanging their back legs from a branch that would place the animal at a height that was easy to work with. Place a pot or some form of contraption under the animal so you can catch all of the blood and unwanted pieces of the animal, as this will help you hide your scent trail later. If you are butchering a squirrel or something of similar size, you can skip the hanging process and just hold the animal upside down over a small bowl. Once you have the animal placed, you will use a sharp knife to slit their throats so that they can bleed out. If your animal is small enough, you can remove the head all at once. If not, wait until it bleeds out and then cut the rest of the head off.

Once the animal has bled out, you will remove the pelt. For small game, you can do this by cutting off all of their feet and their head and then cutting from the inside of one back leg across to the inside of another back leg, so the pelt is separated and then pulling it down toward the head until it is removed. For a medium game, use a sharp knife and cut around the back ankles. Then, cut from one of the ankles to the opposite ankle, running your blade above the tail, so you do not cut into the genital area. Cut off the front feet and the head and tug the pelt down over the head. If your pelt is large enough to be used, cut up one side of it, so it is one flat piece or cut both sides, so you have two parts, and then hang it out to dry by attaching one rope to each corner of the pelt and hanging it, so the pelt is taut.

After the pelt is removed, you will go to the belly side of the animal and make a small incision where their belly button would be, taking caution not to cut into their organs. If you cut into their organs, bile or other digestive enzymes can leach into your meat and render it inedible, so be very careful. Once you have cut a small slit in the belly button, insert your finger and press the organs back, then carefully cut from that slit all the way down to the chest cavity, so you have a large opening over their belly. Next, you will reach into that opening and carefully use your hands to break all of the connective tissues and pull the organs out in front of the animal. Once everything is disconnected and hanging out, you will cut around the genitals to completely remove the intestines from the animal. Throw them away, unless you want to keep the heart and liver, in which case harvest those first and then throw the rest away.

Once your animal has been cut and entrails removed, you can start cutting your pieces. Start by cutting off the front legs and placing them in your consumption container. Then, cut along the spine on either side and remove the flank meat. Lastly, remove meat from the breast area if you have an animal that contained a large amount of breast meat. Then, cut off the back legs and remove the feet if you have not already.

You can also leave your animal intact, not removing any segments of the meat, if you plan on cooking it whole. For animals like squirrels and rabbits, this is perfectly fine as you should have an easy enough time cooking them thoroughly over your fire. For hares or larger animals, however, it is recommended that you cut them down so you can cook them evenly and thoroughly and avoid getting sick from undercooked meat.

Butchering Birds

Butchering birds is different from mammals since they have two legs and wings, and their organs are placed differently than they are for mammals. To butcher a bird, you will need a flat, clean work surface. If you have a table, use that. If not, lay a clean tarp out over a flat spot on the ground and do your butchering there.

You will start the process by first boiling a large pot of water, big enough that you can submerge the entire bird in. As the water warms up, cut the birds head off and let it bleed out into your discard bucket. Then, once the water is warm enough and the bird is bled out, you can hold it by the foot and dip it into the boiling pot of water and move it around. After about 30 seconds, remove the bird and try to pull a feather off of the wing. Keep submerging the bird for about 15 seconds at a time until the wing feathers easily pull off. Once they do, stop submerging the bird and pluck all of the feathers off.

Next, lay the bird on your flat work surface and cut their feet off at the knees. Use your sharp knife to cut the cartilage in the knees, then use your hands to pry the joint apart. Do not use your knife on bones as you will dull it out, and then you will have to sharpen it before you can finish the process. For small birds like doves or quails, you can remove their wings as they are too small to consume. For larger birds like ducks or geese, you can leave them on if you wish.

Once the feet and wings are removed, you will need to remove the neck and gizzards, and then the guts from your bird. Start with the neck. To do so, take your knife and cut around the entire neck area, being careful not to cut into any of the innards. Then, reach in with your hand and remove the innards from your bird. If you are not going to eat the neck and gizzard, throw them into your discard bucket. Next, go to the vent side of the bird, locate the breast bone, and make an incision a few inches below that. Cut carefully around the vent until you reach the tail, and then reach your hands into the incision you have made and gently pull apart all of the connective tissues that hold the organs in place. Pull the organs out as you go, so they are on the outside of your bird. Once you have all of the entrails removed, you can lift them up out of the way and cut beneath the tail, again taking care not to damage any of the organs as you do. At that point, the organs should easily fall out of your bird.

Butchering Fish and Reptiles

Butchering fish and reptiles is different from game and birds because their organs are wildly different from mammals. They are still incredibly easy to butcher, though, and they offer excellent protein when needed.

For fish, you will start by running the back of your knife over your fish to descale it. After you have descaled the fish, cut off the head and tail, and then the fins. Then, take your blade and place it just above the midline of the stomach, by the tail end. Insert your blade most of the way into the fish, but not all the way up through the top spinal area, and slice all the way to the front of the fish. Do this again on the bottom of the midline of the stomach. Once you are done, reach in and pull the midline out, and with it, all of the guts should come out, too. If you have a female fish, the eggs should also be easy to remove at this point, also. You can cook or preserve the fish this way, or when you are ready to cook the fish, you could cut it all the way in half and remove the bones then cook it over your fire.

For reptiles, it depends on what type of reptile you are butchering. Snakes can be slaughtered by cutting off their heads and tails, then descaling and slicing them similar to how you would with a fish, before removing their entrails. For reptiles or amphibians with legs, like lizards or frogs, the process is slightly different. Both lizards and frogs have strong skin, so you will first remove their head and all four feet. Then, you will make an incision into their stomach, cutting through the thick skin. This will take some force, but be careful not to cut too hard, or you will damage the organs, and render the meat useless. Once you have made the incision, you will cut all the way around until you have one large incision around the midsection of the animal. Then, you will tug the skin off the top and bottom, leaving you with a skinned reptile or amphibian. At this point, you can easily remove all of the organs by carefully tugging off the connective tissues and letting the organs fall out of the stomach area, before cutting them away. What's left should be only the edible meat portions of your reptile or amphibian. Because they are so small, there is no need to cut them into sections.

Cleaning and Cooking Wild-Caught Meat

As soon as you are done butchering any sort of wild-caught meat, whether it is a small mammal, bird, fish, or reptile, you need to clean it. Clean your meat by pouring fresh, filtered water over it and ensuring that all of the excess blood, veins, and other little debris are washed away from your meat. Then, get your meat cool as soon as possible. If you have cool water, you can drop your meat into that; if not, you can place it in a tarp and tie it up then float it in a stream of cool water. You want the meat to cool down as soon as possible, so it does not spoil.

When you are ready to cook your meat, you will either place it in a piece of cookware or attach it to a large branch using some form of wire or twine and then you will place it in the low part of the fire, just above the embers. Cook your meat until it is charred on the outside and until it appears overcooked on the inside. It may not taste as good this way, but this will prevent you from accidentally ingesting undercooked meat, which could lead to illness, parasitic infection, or other issues, all of which could be fatal in the bush.

Properly Storing Food

Any food you cannot immediately consume needs to be properly stored. If you are in a snowy area, store leftover food in containers by digging a hole into the snow, burying them, and then marking where they have been buried so you can locate them later on. One way you can store your meat if you do not have snow is by drying it. Slice the meat thin and hang it over fire smoke until it is completely dried out, or let it sit in direct sunlight until it is completely dried out. In this case, you need to cut the meat as thin as possible so you can dry it out quickly, as it could become contaminated if it takes too long. Smoke will both dry the meat out and kill off any bacteria, as smoke is acidic and can protect the meat itself.

Another way to store your meat is to salt it. To do this, you want to coat the meat in salt and then store it in a container. Salt makes the outsides of the meat undesirable to bacteria, as it turns them acidic. You will still need to cook the meat even if you have salt cured it.

Once you have properly cured your meat, you need to place it and your vegetation matter into some form of a bag. You can use a bag you already have, or you can lay everything in the center of a tarp and tie the edges together, so it forms a bag around your food. Then, to safely store your food, you need to hang it from a tree. Hanging your food ensures that no one can get to it, so long as you do it properly. Any other method of storage, such as hiding it or burying it, would lead to your food being dug up and taken by a predator, and it could lead to your cooking camp becoming a dangerous location as predators may come back in search of more.

To hang your food from a tree, you want to find a branch that is high enough that an animal could not reach it from below or above. Understand that large bears can reach as high as six feet, so you need to have your food anchored quite high above the ground. It should also not be anchored anywhere near your camp, or your cooking camp. Keep it at least 100 yards away from your sleeping camp, and 50 yards away from your cooking camp. To anchor it, start by taking a small stick that is around 4 inches long and 2 inches wide and tying a piece of rope around it. This is called a "toggle." Then, toss that over your chosen branch that will be able to keep your food safest. Tie the other end of your rope around the food bag, then simply pull until the food bag is suspended high in the air, but not close to any branches or to the tree trunk of the tree it is hanging from, or any other tree trunk. It should primarily be hanging over a clearing. Then, take the end with the toggle and tie it around the tree, using the toggle to tie it tight and keep it well-fastened in place. Your food should now be safe until you are ready to obtain it for consumption later on. Anytime you come back for your food, be particularly aware of any predators, as the fact that they cannot access your food does not mean that they will not be attracted to the area. They may linger around, trying to look for a way to access it, so you need to be extra cautious to avoid accidentally walking up on a hungry predator.

Long-Term Gardening Solutions

If you are in the wilderness for an extended period of time, you need to start learning how to garden. Long-term gardening solutions ensure that you have a plentiful supply of fresh produce for as long as you need it. Gardening can be done by foraging for seeds from local flora, or you can pack seeds of the hardiest plants for your survival area's hardiness zone in your G'n'G bag for just in case. If you do this, be sure to update your seeds from time to time as they will go dormant and die eventually if they are not used.

The best way to engage in a long-term gardening solution in the wilderness is to build raised bed gardens and forage for soil from the local area to fill your raised bed gardens with. Large branches off of trees can easily be used to build your gardens, as can larger rocks. Once your bed is filled, you can place your seeds in it and tend to it as you would with a regular garden. The benefit here is that you have access to a consistent crop and that you can consume food without having to go searching for it all the time. However, you will need to be cautious as omnivores and herbivores like deer, mice, rabbits, and other animals may find your garden and start eating it. While this may seem like a great way to get your hands on more animal protein, it is also a great way to lose access to your abundant garden. You may need to build some form of fence or protection to keep your garden safe so no one can steal it from you.

CHAPTER 9

The Fifth Essential: Safety

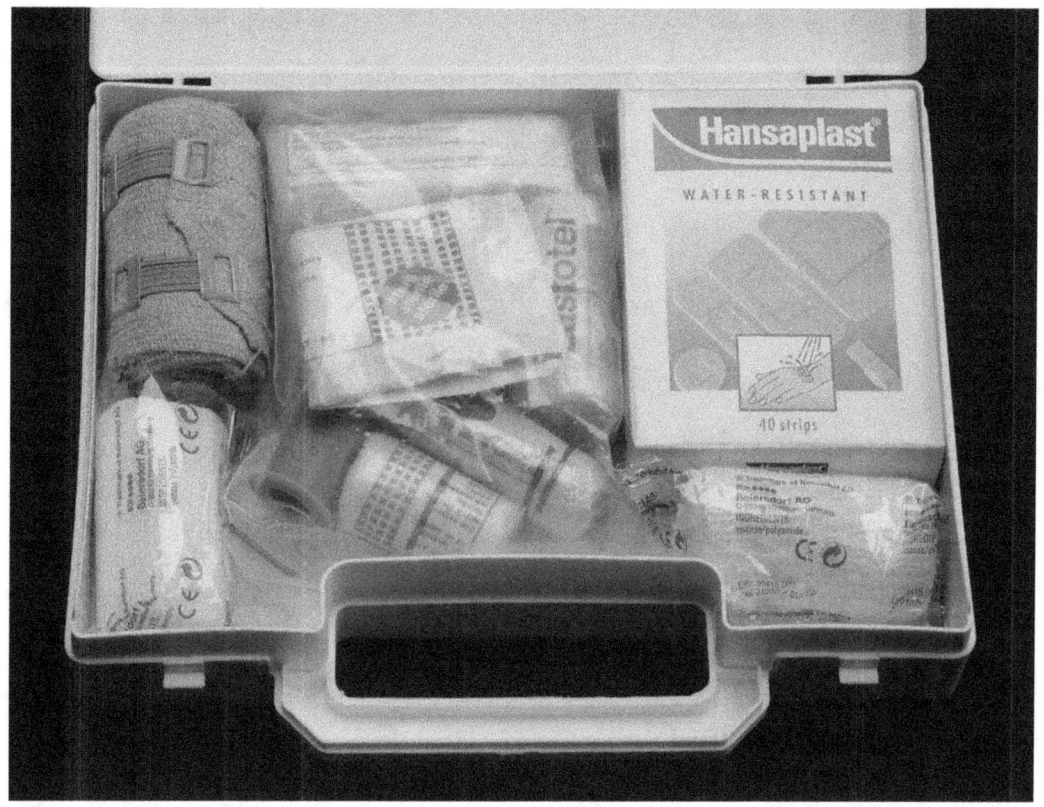

Safety is an essential part of survival, as unsafe conditions can lead to accidental illness, injury, or death. Your mental, emotional, and physical health are all at risk when you are unable to maintain your safety, as you will find yourself living in constant fear and likely being harmed by the dangers around you. The better you protect yourself, the longer you can survive. It is essential that you cover all safety bases, and that you do not take any for granted, as a lack of safety in any area of your life can lead to serious side effects.

At home, practicing safety seems standard and is often considered a form of common sense. For example, don't touch a hot stove, never leave a gas burner on unattended, or don't fall asleep in the bathtub. In the bush, safety can be far more challenging to navigate because you are not entirely aware of what the dangers are or how they could affect you. Another aspect of safety that many people do not realize is how much easier it is to get sick in the bush. At home, your environment is usually sterile, and if it isn't, you have immediate access to first aid equipment or a doctor if one is needed. This means that if you get sick or injured, you have a sterile environment to get better in, or if you need access to medical care you have a trained professional to help you.

There are many more risks in the wilderness you may not be aware of, as well as far fewer sterilization guidelines and medical experts who can help you navigate sickness or injury. Learning how to keep your environment as clean as possible, practice essential hygiene steps to keep yourself clean and safe, and know how to handle first aid situations, so you are less likely to find yourself in a dangerous situation. This way, if anything does go wrong, you know how to navigate it, and you can navigate it quickly.

Rather than attempting to rely on the common sense that keeps you safe in an urban environment, it is critical that you educate yourself on the real harms of the wilderness and how you can protect yourself from those harms. The more you can protect yourself, the better.

Protecting Yourself From Predators

The first and possibly most obvious safety risk you need to be aware of in the bush is predators. Aside from the already-known widowmakers, predators are also an issue. Predators are often viewed as being large, obviously aggressive mammals such as bears, wolves, or other animals that are routinely depicted in movies as the dangers of the wilderness. The reality is, there are far more predators in the wilderness than you are likely aware of. Foxes, coyotes, bobcats, lynx, cougars, and other large animals are all considered predators. Even smaller mammals like badgers, wolverines, and Tasmanian devils are all wildly dangerous and can cause harm to you. If you come across a moose, a buck, or any male species of animal that has horns such as elk, antelope, mountain goats, or otherwise, you may also be at risk. Especially during mating season, these animals can be quite dangerous and will use their antlers or horns to attack you, and they can cause fatal injuries in minimal timing.

From the ground, venomous spiders, bugs, and reptiles are all risks you need to be aware of. One bite from a venomous animal could lead to serious illness and injury, and some can even lead to death within a matter of hours. Poisonous frogs with toxins in their skin can lead to delirium, among other forms of sickness, both neurological and physical. Even something as simple as a mosquito infected with an illness can be fatal if it bites you, and you become infected with that illness. You must be aware of the fact that predators are not always large, obvious mammals that have big teeth and menacing claws. In fact, many predators don't look like that at all. You must be aware of what is around you and always focus on keeping distance between yourself and other living beings. Even if something seems harmless, stay away. You never know what it is carrying, or how it may affect you.

The most obvious way to protect yourself from predators is to stay away from them. However, that may not always be enough. Keeping a large knife on hand and within reach is always a good idea, as it gives you direct access to a weapon that you can use should you need to fight off an animal physically. Throwing rocks and sticks at an animal, yelling at them, and staying near fire is a great way to protect yourself. If you lack tools for protection, you need to make yourself seem bigger and scarier than the animal that is taunting you, as this prevents them from trying to attack you. If you do have tools like bear mace, use them. However, you should beware that this may not always work on all species of animals.

Another way to keep yourself safe is to keep your shoes tightly tied, tuck in your clothes so insects cannot get into them, and keep your sleeping bag wrapped tightly around you to avoid making an entrance for insects. As well, before ever getting into your shelter, sleeping bag, or any other sit down or lie down location, or enclosed space, always look for possible threats. Keep an eye out for reptiles, bugs, and small animals that may have gotten in, and safely remove them before entering yourself. This way, you are less likely to encounter an accidental bite, scratch, or other injuries that could quickly turn into a serious issue.

Keeping Yourself and Your Camp Hygienic

Hygiene is one of the most important things you can focus on in the bush. A lack of hygiene can rapidly lead to illness, either by you consuming a bacteria that makes you ill or by a seemingly minor wound becoming infected. Even scratches you cannot see with the naked eye can become infected with a staph infection, or worse, and can turn into a serious health hazard. You must keep yourself and your space hygienic at all times to avoid having any harmful bacteria introduced to your system so that your body is able to remain fit and abled for as long as it needs to be.

To keep yourself and your camp hygienic, you need to consider the likely areas where bacteria would exist and routinely sterilize them to keep them as free of bacteria as possible. This includes obvious things such as cookware and hunting tools, and less obvious things such as your clothes, your mouth, and your skin. Even your bed should be routinely sterilized to prevent bacteria from building up and causing sickness.

The first thing you need to keep hygienic is yourself. One of the most important things that many people do not realize is the importance of keeping your feet dry. You must always have a dry pair of socks and footwear on at all times. Wet feet can blister, and chronically wet feet can develop fungal infections, and those infections are nearly impossible to treat in the bush unless you have the right tools. If your infections last too long, they can turn into wounds that can become gangrenous and can cause you to die. It does not take nearly as long to reach that point as you would think, either, since you are in an area where it is challenging to maintain a truly sterile environment.

Aside from your feet, it is also important that the rest of you remain dry, too. While your feet are most at-risk, the rest of your body can develop issues if you are constantly wet, also. On wet days, stay indoors as much as possible and let yourself fully dry out before going back out to complete any chores, so your body is not constantly wet. If you can, wear layers that will prevent your skin from getting wet at all. In a dire scenario, you could make a rain poncho out of a tarp, or even out of an animal hide or a few animal hides sewn together if you need one.

Keeping your mouth sterile is important, also. Your mouth comes into contact with large amounts of bacteria, all of which are usually eliminated when you brush your teeth. If you do not have a proper toothbrush and toothpaste to clean your teeth with, you will want to drink plenty of water after each meal and swish your mouth out several times a day to keep bacteria out of your mouth. You can also look for a dogwood or sassafras tree and take some of the inner bark from that tree, then chew on it. They will become highly fibrous, and both are high in tannic acid, which is an effective antibacterial agent. You could also make a tea with dogwood or sassafras bark and use it as an antiseptic mouthwash as needed.

To keep your body clean, the best way is through smoke baths. Every time you have a campfire, be sure to intentionally stand in the smoke so your body and hair can be sterilized. Make sure you take your clothes off and do this to your naked body, as well, so your entire body is staying clean. Smoke baths are particularly useful as they will help hide your natural odor, too, which means animals are less likely to detect your scent. This means you can stay hidden longer and acts like hunting will be much easier since you will not have a distinct odor that the animals can pick up on. You can also hang your clothes and bedding in a smoky area so they take on the smoke, as this can also help keep them clean. Hang them in direct sunlight for at least two hours, too, as sunlight can kill of virtually any bacteria that may linger on them.

Keeping your hands clean in the bush is best done by finding a yucca plant, yarrow, or another plant in your area that is high in saponins. You cannot ingest saponins as they are poisonous; however, they are also known for killing off bacteria. Necessarily, saponins are soap. To use it, take a piece of the plant and get it wet and then rub it vigorously between your hands. Your hands will then be clean.

For your camp, you need to ensure that you start with the basics. Keep blood and other visible contaminants off of everything, and sterilize anything that comes into contact with blood using boiling hot water. If something, like a sewing needle, needs to come into contact with the body or a wound, ensure it is passed through fire several times or boiled first to kill off any bacteria that may be lingering. In your first aid kit you can also keep some antibacterial wipes. However, you should refrain from using those except for in dire situations as you do not want to run out of them in a low-importance situation and find yourself in need of them in something that takes higher priority.

You can also keep your camp clean by keeping everything separated. Keep hygiene products, clothing, bedding, footwear, cookware, trapping and fishing gear, safety tools, and everything else separated so that if something does become contaminated, it is more challenging for it to contaminate anything else. Wash your hands regularly when going between different things, so you are not picking up or spreading germs around. You can also routinely expose your tools and belongings to sunlight for at least two hours, as the sunlight will help kill any contaminants. Do not reuse clothes, dishes, or tools without cleaning in between as they can begin to build up with bacteria, and this can lead to illnesses being introduced to your camp.

Although you cannot perfectly clean your camp environment, do your best to keep it free of objects that may be hazardous. Remove sharp branches, sticks, and rocks, keep the ground area clean, and keep everything as organized as possible. Keep a shovel handy, and any time you have to go to the bathroom, be sure to do it at least 50-100 yards away from camp, and bury it every time. This way, you are not exposed to possible bacteria in your urine or feces, which could lead to you becoming sick and transmitting sickness to others. Doing this will also keep predators away because it will hide any scents that could attract wildlife that may be coming from your camp.

Lastly, you should have a specific first aid location that can be used for helping anyone who has fallen ill or becomes injured in any way. This location should be kept clean and organized, and absolutely nothing should take place in this location unless it is first aid related. If you can, keep a sterile tarp folded up and lay that over the first aid location before treating anything, so you are less likely to introduce or pick up any bacteria from your first aid location. It is extremely important that you are very careful about anything getting into or around your wound when you are wounded in the bush, as even a small introduction of a harmful bacteria can be fatal. Be vigilant, stay clean, and do everything you can to keep bacteria away from you and your camp members.

First Aid Skills You Need to Know

Keeping a proper first aid kit available in your camp is essential. The first aid kit should never be touched or opened unless it is actually needed. When it is opened, it should be done so carefully and by someone who has washed their hands and is in as clean of an environment as possible to prevent them from introducing bacteria to the first aid kit. There are four major first aid skills you need to have in the bush, which will allow you to navigate nearly any emergency you may face: how to treat burns, how to dress wounds, how to set broken bones, and how to deal with illness.

Treating Burns

Accidents around fires can rapidly lead to burns, and improper treatment can lead to serious wounds that can cause nasty life-threatening infections, as well as harsh scarring. Treating burns promptly and properly is essential when it comes to keeping yourself or the affected individual safe.

The first thing to do is to stop the burning process. Even if the heat has been removed from the area, the skin itself will still be burning, so you need to stop this process. If you have cool filtered water, carefully run it over the burn. If not, you need to cover the burn and submerge the arm into cool water without having the water get into the burn itself to avoid contamination with bacteria or parasites.

If you can, elevate the burn to reduce swelling that could be sustained from the burn injury. Then, cover the area lightly with a non-stick dressing like sterile gauze, not cotton or adhesive bandages. If you can, you need to seek medical treatment immediately. If you cannot, you need to monitor the burn. It is likely that it will remain red, blister, and turn into a wound. At that point, you can start following wound protocol to keep the burn clean and to treat the resulting wound. If the burn reaches this point, it is likely that scarring will occur.

Dressing Wounds

Dressing wounds is important, as you need to know how to properly clean the area, treat it, and keep it covered to prevent harmful bacteria from being introduced. If you have a deeper wound, you want to let it bleed for a few minutes as the blood rushing out of the wound will push any bacteria out, too. However, you do not want to let the bleeding go on for a prolonged period of time, as this could lead to other issues related to excessive blood loss.

After a few seconds and no more than about two or three minutes, depending on the severity of bleeding (shorter bleed time for more aggressive bleeding), you need to stop the bleeding. Using gauze or your cleanest t-shirt, place it over the wound and press firmly to stop blood flow. This should allow it to begin coagulating so it can stop actively bleeding out of the wound. If you can, raise the wound above heart level, as this will make it easier for it to stop bleeding. Pressure should be applied for at least 10 minutes to stop the bleeding. If it isn't stopping the bleeding, you may need to insert your fingers, locate the severed vein or artery, and apply pressure this way to stop the bleeding.

Next, you need to clean the wound. Do this by removing the dressing for a few moments and flushing the wound with filtered drinking water from 1-2 inches away, at an angle perpendicular to the wound. You should use at least 8 ounces of water, though you may need more if the wound is covered in dirt and debris from the injury itself.

Now you need to assess the wound and decide how to cover it. Scrapes will not be able to be pulled back together, so covering them with a sterile bandage is the best option. Ripped skin, animal bites, or punctures can often be pulled back together using duct tape, stitch-style bandages, or sutures. You may also be able to superglue them together if you have access to this in your kit but only do this if it is a clean cut; otherwise, it could cause you to seal bacteria inside the wound. If an injury looks more like a chunk has been removed, you will need to moisten gauze with potable water and pack the wound with it before dressing it so that nothing can get into the wound.

Lastly, you need to dress the wound. To do this, moisten a pad with antibiotic ointment and place it over the wound. Then, cover it with a dry pad, and finally use self-adhesive tape or something similar to keep the pads in place. Now, you need to get medical help as soon as possible, if possible, because life-threatening infections can set in, in as little as six hours.

Setting Broken Bones

Broken bones in the woods can be highly dangerous. They make it so you are unable to reasonably navigate the woods, and they can leave you at risk of malformation if the bone does not heal properly, or illness if the wound becomes infected during the healing process. If a broken bone has occurred in the head, neck, or back, the only course of action is to stabilize the person and get help immediately, do not try to move the person because it could result in further damage.

If the bone is sticking out of the skin, if the bleeding will not stop or is spurting like a fountain, or if there is a loss of feeling or warmth at or beyond the injured area, prompt medical attention is also required. There is no safe way to treat this level of trauma in the bush, as the affected individual can die from either shock, improperly set bones, or infection getting deep into the body through the wound.

The first thing you must do with any broken bone is stop the bleeding, if there is bleeding occurring. If there is any bone sticking out or pushing through the skin, do not try to touch it or push it back in place as you could cause serious damage in the process. After the bleeding has stopped, you need to splint the area if possible. At this point, you want to remove any clothing from the area and apply the splint directly to the affected limb, though you do not want to move the broken bone, so if you have to, you need to cut the clothes away from the break. Then, you need to gently tape the fractured bone to a rolled-up piece of paper, a stick, or a rolled-up piece of clothing that will help keep the bone more stable. The joint above and below should be included in the splint if possible. Never try to force or twist the limb back into place, and never try to move it unless it is absolutely necessary because doing so could cause further injury.

Next, you need to do what you can to reduce swelling and prevent further injury to the place by applying an ice pack and elevating the injury if possible. If you have any, you can administer ibuprofen, acetaminophen, or naproxen. Do not give aspirin to anyone under 18 years old. As soon as you can, get medical attention, as broken bones are not easily managed in the wilderness.

Dealing With Illness

Illness can strike for many reasons, and during a survival situation, you could be at higher risk of falling ill due to the fact that you are stressed, and your body is struggling to cope with the stress. When you fall ill in the bush, you need to treat your symptoms as soon as possible, as illness can rapidly become dangerous. For example, if you have diarrhea or are vomiting, you could become seriously dehydrated in as little as twelve to twenty-four hours. If you have a stomach ache, your inability to eat could lead to additional symptoms caused by your lack of incoming nutrients when your body needs them most. Even a headache can be difficult, as headaches can make getting daily tasks done far more challenging and can leave you unable to acquire the resources you need. Further, when you are ill, it is far more challenging to mask your scent and protect yourself from predators, which leaves you especially vulnerable.

In the wilderness, treating these conditions requires you to sip potable water as often as possible. You can also take some charcoal from the bottom of the fire and drink it in a glass of water, though you do not want to drink too much as this would not be good. A small teaspoon in a glass of water can help flush any toxins out of your digestive system, though it may cause you to experience more diarrhea and vomiting for a short period of time as the toxins are being flushed out. Sipping tea made of sassafras, yarrow, brambles, nettles, plantain, ground ivy, cleavers, clover, or mallow can also help settle an upset stomach to prevent further diarrhea or vomiting.

If you have a headache, sipping tea made from willow bark can be helpful, as willow bark is said to be nature's aspirin. It contains analgesic properties that help reduce pain, making it easier for you to get over a painful headache or even dull aches in your body from days of hard work.

Foraging for Medicinal Plants

Foraging for plants that have medicinal value is similar to foraging for plants that you can consume. The safest way to do so is to have a foraging book designed for your unique geographical location, and that contains valuable information that shows you what to forage, and how, and that shows you how to avoid foraging for the wrong thing. As well, foraging with a local herbalist or wildcrafter is a great idea as they are trained in the local flora. These professionals can show you what the medicinal plants are in your location, where to find them, and how to use them.

CHAPTER 10

The Great Escape

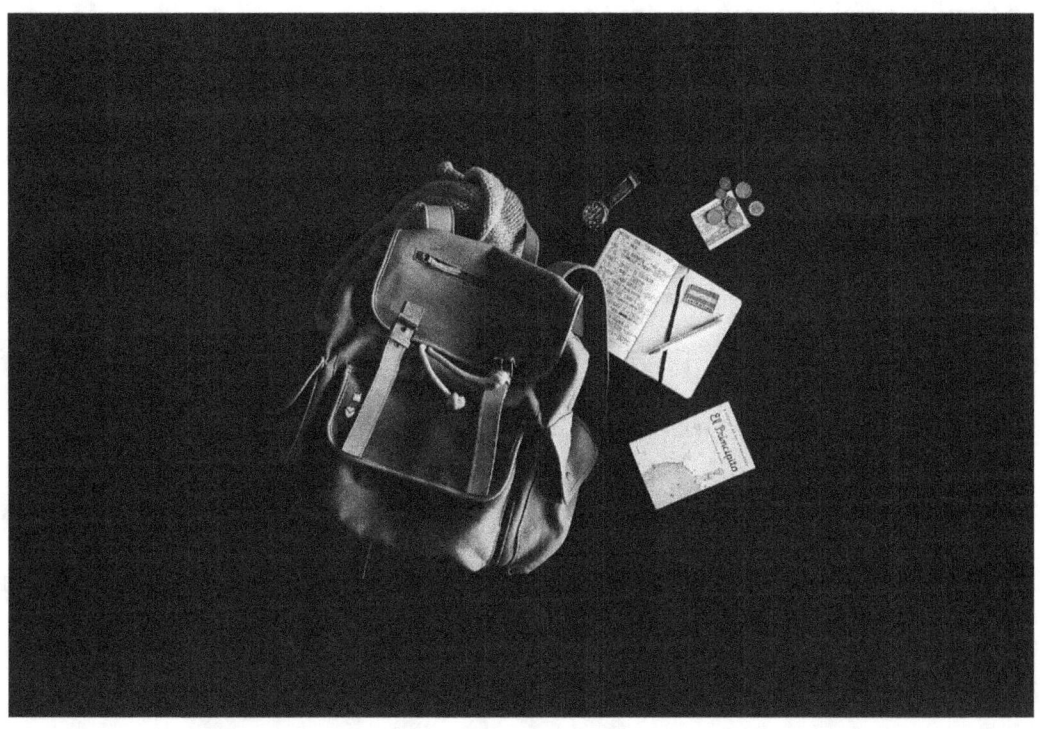

Knowing how to escape when escape is needed is as important as knowing how to survive once you have already escaped. One wrong step during your escape could lead to you and your family being exposed to even greater dangers, or possibly dying due to the impending threat, because you took a wrong step. Often, emergencies require careful consideration and approaches, two things that are extremely hard to navigate when you are already highly stressed out. As soon as you become stressed out, your body naturally slips into fight or flight response, or worse, freeze or faint. At this point, convincing yourself to do anything may seem challenging, including escaping an emergency situation. The best way to prepare yourself for any escape, whether you need to escape indoors or escape to the wilderness, is to rehearse what needs to happen and engage in repetition by reminding yourself of the process over and over again. This way, when the emergency strikes, hopefully, your instinct kicks in, and you follow those repeated patterns and get yourself, and your family, safely removed from the emergency.

Escaping Minor Emergencies

Escaping minor emergencies requires you to escape the immediate vicinity of danger. Most minor emergencies will not require more than maybe 100 feet to 100 yards of space between yourself and the emergency to keep yourself safe. For example, if you are inside your house and a fire breaks out, you need to escape to the outdoors. Alternatively, if you are outside of your house and a thunderstorm strikes or a heavy windstorm kicks up, you need to get indoors.

Escaping a minor emergency truly depends on what emergency you are escaping, and what sort of threat that emergency poses. If you need to escape your house, you should have several clear escape routes planned so that you can run away from the danger, while safely bringing your family with you. This way, if something were to happen like a fire or a dangerous flood, you could quickly remove yourself from your house.

If you need to escape into your house, you should have a plan for where you will go. For example, in the event of a serious storm, you want to get indoors and stay away from possible hazards. Often, this means staying away from windows, doors, and open fireplaces with chimneys. If you are facing a serious windstorm or a tornado, you want to get to the lowest floor in your house and hide as far away from any heavy furniture as possible, as well as away from windows, doors, and fireplaces with chimneys. Your furnace, electrical wires, and gas lines also need to be inspected as even seemingly small or non-observed disasters can damage these, and they can be life-threatening.

Escaping Major Emergencies

If you are in a major emergency and you need to escape your city, you must be ready to escape safely. Prepare for your escape with a full tank of gas in your vehicle or with arrangements to meet up with someone who has a vehicle and can help you escape if you do not drive. You should also have your G'n'G bags packed and ready to go. Your larger bags may be at home, but you should have smaller bags with you in your car at all times so that if you have to escape and cannot return home first, you can escape with what you have and still have at least a few things to help you get started.

As soon as you have everything and are on the road, you need to take the most direct route out of the city as you possibly can. The route may be thick with people also trying to escape, so be patient and move as quickly as you can without risking yourself or anyone else, as car accidents are not ideal at this point in time. For some emergencies, it can be particularly scary. For example, in some cases, people are driving away from their hometowns while wildfires are on the side of the road they are driving on, or are driving away just hours before a major hurricane is due to hit. Either way, you need to be as patient as possible.

It is important to understand that when you are escaping from your city, there is a time to leave, and then there is a time to stay. You need to leave early enough that you actually have time to escape, even with all of the gridlock that may be happening on local roads. Otherwise, you might find yourself in even more danger as you are trapped in your car when disaster strikes. It is vital that you listen to emergency warnings and that you heed those warnings as soon as possible. With any luck, you escape well enough in advance that you are safe, and you can stay with friends or family elsewhere who are not set to be affected by the disaster. If the disaster is a pandemic or the enforcement of a police state, it may make more sense to skip trying to stay with anyone and instead head to the wilderness to set up camp and keep to yourself until everything becomes safer.

If you must stay, or if you escape, but without enough time, you will likely find yourself facing a disaster where you have to embrace your wilderness skills to protect yourself and your family. In this case, the first step for escaping is to keep yourself safe while the disaster strikes. Find somewhere safe to be, such as a storm cellar, or somewhere that is covered with a steady, strong building that is unlikely to collapse. Avoid hiding around vehicles, under trees, near furniture that could fall down, near windows or doors, or on the level of a house that has the roof in case the roof is damaged in the storm. If heavy flooding is present, without wind storms or lightning, you may need to get to higher ground either by heading to the highest floor in your house or even getting up onto your roof to stay away from the flooding. Weather the storm using your G'n'G bag and listening to updates that will inform you as to what is going on and what you can do to keep yourself safe. Always pay close attention to radio updates, as authorities will let you know what you can do to stay safe and will use the radio to broadcast where you can go or how you can get relief if you are trapped or in need of rescuing.

Once the disaster is done, you need to assess the damage and decide your course of action. If you are able to safely stay in your home location, you can stay there. Otherwise, you may need to commence your escape once the storm has passed so that you can either go stay elsewhere or stay in the wilderness in a safer location until it is safer for you to return home.

CHAPTER 11

The Unspoken Essential Of Survival

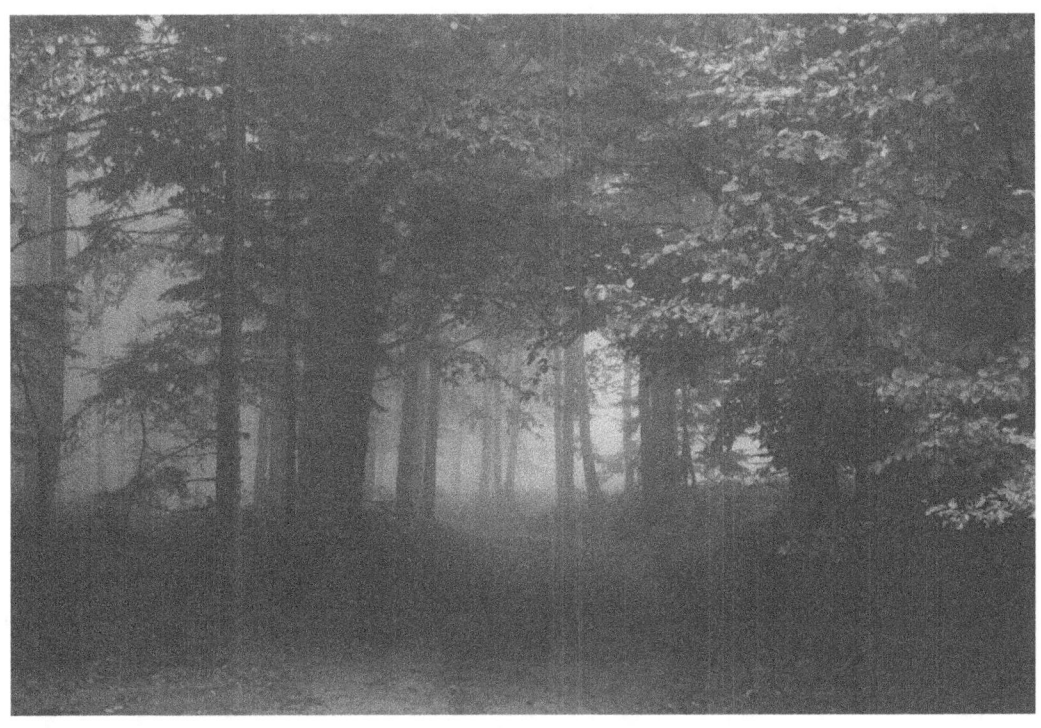

One unspoken essential of survival that almost no one talks about also happens to be one of the most influential aspects of your survival. In fact, if you do not manage this particular aspect of your survival, you can completely lose the ability to survive and may find yourself floundering or even dying in a situation where it may have been perfectly feasible to survive. If you watch any of the reality shows on TV that focus on survival skills, you likely already know what this unspoken essential of survival is, as many of the contestants on those shows come across it and find themselves quitting prematurely. That is, your mindset.

If you are in the wilderness, your mindset must be focused on survival, as a mindset focused on anything else can lead to distractions and increased challenges placed on your survival. Focusing on everything going wrong, rather than everything you can do to protect yourself, elevates your stress, and makes necessary survival techniques far more challenging. Some people in real survival situations will even die because of the stress itself. In many cases of rescue missions where entire groups were stranded, there have been instances where one or two people passed away either due to suicide or due to a lack of will to survive, which ultimately cost them their lives. You *must* learn how to strengthen your will and reinforce your mindset if you are going to survive dangerous situations. Without your mindset on board, predators and nasty bacteria are minor dangers in comparison to what you are up against.

The Biggest Danger Lurking At Two AM

In the wilderness, there is a time of day that is known as being the darkest hour. That is, at two AM. All day long, survivalists are focused on fulfilling tasks essential to their survival and are playing an active role in their wellbeing, and the wellbeing of those they are stranded with. This active role results in them feeling as though they have some sense of control over their situation, and like all will be okay because they are able to keep themselves going. Unfortunately, at two AM, there is no active role. You are supposed to be sleeping. You may have even been sleeping until something woke you up.

Once you are awake, it is easy for the reality of what you are going through to set in, and with nothing to keep you active or busy, it can be challenging to move those thoughts out of your mind. On reality TV, countless conversations about these hardships and giving up have been recorded and shared for thousands to see. What people don't realize is that off of reality TV, in real survival settings, thousands more of these conversations have actually happened, and many have ended in people not surviving to see the next day, or not surviving through to see the rescue mission.

At 2 AM, when everything else is calm, you must focus on one thing, and one thing only: getting back to sleep. Your body needs your rest, and you need the break from everything you are up against. Allowing yourself to stay awake, pondering the many things you are facing will only lead to you feeling a greater sense of stress and burden, which will ultimately drive you into the depths of depression and anxiety. For some people, hysteria sets in, and that in and of itself can be a highly dangerous place to be in.

It may seem like an impossible discipline to reel your mind back into a state of control, but it is essential if you are going to survive. You need to learn how to shut down thoughts, refuse to entertain your fears, and focus exclusively on the survival mission at hand. Until you are rescued, your only job is to get from one day to the next, one hour to the next, or one minute to the next, whatever you can handle.

Most people never come across such intense survival experiences in their lives. As a result, they are totally unprepared for the serious mental strength it takes, and for the dangers that can be lurking in their thoughts. If you have never had to withstand this, then you can consider yourself lucky. However, one day you might have to endure it, and if you do, you need to be ready for that 2 AM dread. Being aware of it in advance can help you realize that what you are thinking and feeling is normal, and can help you switch into refusing the thoughts and going back to sleep because you know that this is the healthiest choice you can make. Even if you don't know when you will be rescued, or if you have lost so much, your job is not to focus on that now. Your job is to focus on survival, and the rest can come later. 2 AM is never the right time to sort through your thoughts or your problems. Go to sleep.

Keeping Yourself on Track for Survival

People who survive the wilderness share one thing in common: survival mode. They fiercely click into survival mode and do not stop to question themselves or their actions, because they know they must take them. This lessens their emotional stress and increases their ability to take necessary action for survival. They are worried solely about surviving every single day, period. As a result, their body is able to kick into survival mode with them, and they end up surviving virtually anything they come up against, short of a freak accident or a tragic illness or injury in the bush, which leads to their death.

If you are in the bush, you have to remember that as a human, you are a part of the animal kingdom. Just like every other animal in that bush, you have access to a powerful instinct inside of you that will tell you what to do, where to look, how to move, where to go, and how to keep yourself and anyone else with you alive. Even if you have no idea what you are doing, if you lean into that instinct, it will help you out a lot more than you may expect. Even though we live our modern lives extremely different from the animals in the bush, we are still animals, and we are not nearly as far removed from our instincts as people tend to believe we are.

As soon as you allow yourself to lean into that survival, you will notice that all of your priorities change. Rather than worrying about the past or the future, as humans often do, you will be solely worried about the present. Your instincts will sharpen as your awareness heightens, your ability to navigate difficult terrain is increased, and your understanding of how to survive in the bush seems to come naturally. You will easily spot threats that come your way, you will seemingly "know" how to handle difficult situations, and you will know how to shut out the challenging emotions and keep yourself focused.

In survival mode, none of the emotions matter anymore; only your survival does. You can worry about snapping out of it and healing from all of this later on when the chance arrives. For now, just focus on surviving.

CHAPTER 12

Getting Help When Needed

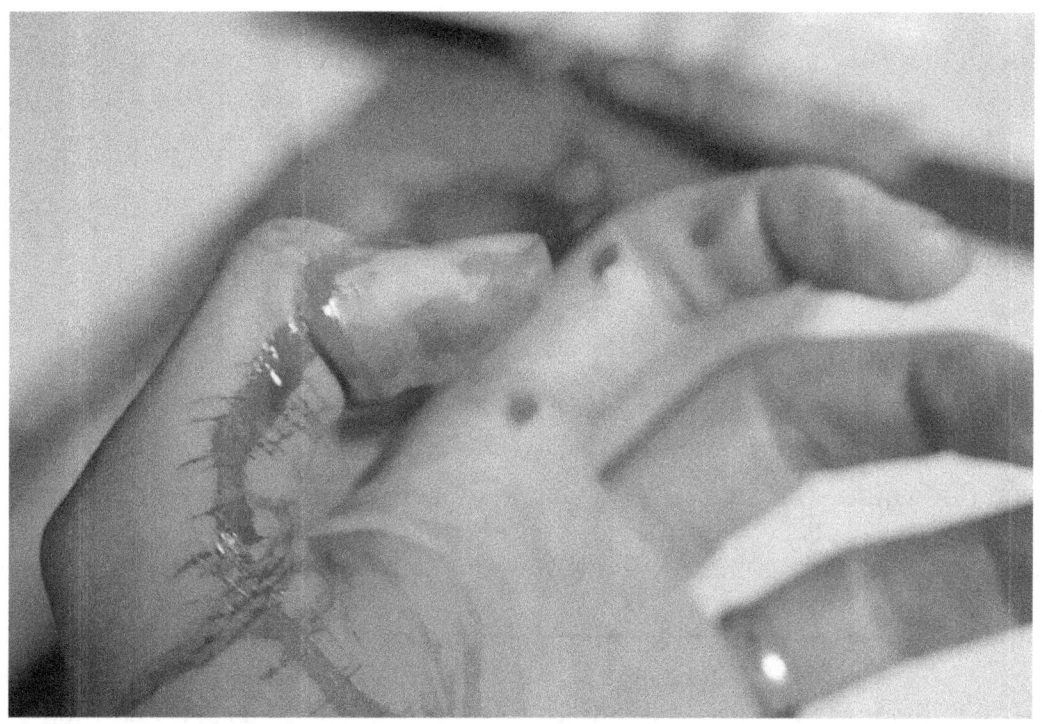

When you are in a survival setting, there are times when you will need to call for help, and times when you won't. Knowing how to determine when is the right time to call, and who to call, is important as it will ensure that you get access to the safety you need as soon as possible. It is also important to understand what needs to be done after calling for help to ensure that anyone who might be coming to help you knows where to find you, what they need to help you, and how to get the job done. The more you can prepare your rescuers for what they are coming to, the easier it will be for them to rescue you safely.

When Is the Right Time to Call?

Knowing when to call for help is important. Amid an emergency situation, it may be hard to determine when you should make that call, or if a call even needs to be made in the first place. For some people, the minute they begin to feel panic, they begin to dial for help, even though that may not be necessary. For others, they might try to engage in a rescue mission alone without calling for help because they don't think there is time, or the emergency itself causes them to completely forget that help is available. Both calling for help when none is needed, or forgetting or refusing to call for help when it is needed, are bad situations to be in.

When you find yourself in an emergency, it is important to pause and ask yourself a few questions about what is going on right now. Is it reasonable for you to navigate this emergency on your own? Or is this something that would be better left to professionals? This may be obvious if you are in a situation where someone has scraped their knee, or where your house is on fire. With a scraped knee, you can easily manage that yourself with your first aid kit, whereas when your house is on fire, it is obvious that you need to call 911. But what if your emergency is something like a serious cut that is bleeding or a severed digit? When it comes to serious emergencies, you must ask yourself how reasonable it is for you to handle this emergency on your own, versus calling for help.

If the injured or affected individual is stable, despite their injury, you may be able to drive them to the hospital yourself. If you can, do this, as it will relieve pressure on emergency services and will also help you save the money it costs to hire emergency transportation services. Further, driving directly to the hospital yourself is faster than having someone drive all the way to your house then to the hospital, even if they are speeding. If the person is not stable or cannot be stabilized, call for help. This means if someone is drowning, if someone has been knocked unconscious and is not waking up, if they are too weak to move, or if it would be dangerous or extremely challenging for you to move them, you call for help.

In some cases, you may be able to rely on the help of a doctor's appointment, or on a simple call to your doctor's office to ensure that you have handled things properly. For example, if you get food poisoning and are quite sick, but are not dehydrated, you can call your doctor or book an appointment without having to call an emergency line. These types of emergencies do need to be handled the right way, but they are not so pressing that you have to call for immediate help.

Always be sure to call the right level of help for your situation, because calling the wrong level of help could lead to you tying up precious resources, having unnecessary expenses to pay, and possibly wasting people's time. Alternatively, not calling the right level of help for your situation could lead to the person who has been affected to fail to receive the necessary level of care that they require. As a result, they could become further injured or ill because the rescue team was ill prepared to deal with the specific situation you are facing.

Who Is the Right Person to Call?

Knowing the right person to call is important. When you are in an emergency, it can be challenging to know who to call as you will be experiencing a great deal of stress and that stress can make navigating your situation seemingly impossible. For this reason, it can be helpful to have a list of specific emergency contacts and numbers you can call in any range of emergencies, as this list will help you know exactly who to call for any given situation. You should keep this list in your G'n'G bag, and another in your car. Keep it laminated or otherwise protected so that if you need it, you are not at risk of grabbing the paper only to find out it has been torn, smudged, or otherwise damaged.

The emergency numbers you should have on hand include any in case of emergency contacts that are relevant to your family, such as your spouse, parents, siblings, or other family members.

You should also have the numbers for:

- Local fire department
- Local police department (non-emergency line)
- C
- oast guard
- Family doctor
- Nurse line
- Nearby hospitals

- Local EMS
- Poison control
- Veterinarian
- Water company
- Power company
- Tow truck
- Animal control
- Locksmith
- Next door neighbors
- Insurance agent
- Important co-workers
- Boss
- Important family members

These numbers are all people you might have to call in an emergency, and having their numbers readily written down means you do not have to go looking for them when the time comes. This can also help you discover the right person to call right away, as you can gauge the level of emergency and call the appropriate number. For example, if you or your family member is experiencing symptoms of possible illness, you could call your family doctor to book an appointment. If they are showing symptoms of illness that cannot wait for an appointment, you can call your local nurse line. If they are showing even bigger symptoms, you can call the hospital and bring them in to be checked. Or, if they are showing symptoms that are so bad that you cannot get them to the hospital yourself, you can call for EMS. Always gauge your call appropriately and call the right people, so you have the right help for the job, as this is key to navigating any emergency quickly and with success. Calling the wrong people could result in you not having the right help that is needed, and that could lead to the emergency growing or becoming more serious as time passes. In emergencies, time is of the essence, so be quick, be accurate, and call for help when you need it.

How Can You Prepare to Be Rescued?

Calling for help may require some preparation on your end when it comes to readying yourself to be rescued. There are different preparation methods required depending on what you are doing, so you want to make sure you have everything you need for your rescue mission on hand.

If you are at home and need rescuing, make sure you are in a place where your rescuers can easily locate you. Be clear about where you are, what help is needed, and how they can find you. In the instance of a house fire or damage to the inside of your home, get outside and wait on the lawn or sidewalk for the rescue team to arrive, so they do not have to rescue you from indoors. If you cannot escape, tell your rescue team where you are so they can quickly access you and remove you from the dangerous location. If you are dealing with something like a serious injury or illness, make sure doors are unlocked, and rescuers know to come in if they can, move the affected individual to the front door if possible, or have someone ready to answer the door when they arrive.

In an outdoor emergency, such as if you are surviving in the wilderness, you may need to find your way to a clearing, to a major road, or to some other form of landmark that is easily accessible by rescuers so you can be rescued. While rescue teams can retrieve you from virtually anywhere because of the high tech gear they carry, it is easier for them to rescue you if you are in an area where they can quickly gain access to. As you wait for your rescue team to come find you, try to get to a clearing or a large landmark, and let your rescue team know that this is your plan. Let them know where you are leaving from, too, so they know where they can find you if you do not make it to the clearing. Never go anywhere that your rescuers do not know you are going, and always tell them where you have been, where you are coming from, and where you are heading. This way, you are able to be saved quicker. If you use a device that GPS pings your location to your rescue team, *do not leave that location*. Even if it is not optimal for being rescued, it is where the rescue team knows to find you, and if you leave that location, they will not be able to find you. *Stay there.*

Is There Ever a Time When You Should Not Call?

There are certain times when you should *not* call for help, even if you are in need of some form of help. The most important one to consider is relevant when you are in a large-scale emergency, but you may not be in a pressing emergency yourself. For example, let's say your town gets hit by a hurricane, and your neighborhood was affected. Perhaps your house has been damaged, or someone in your family has sustained a minor injury, but it is something you can deal with from home. In this case, you should not be in a rush to call for help as doing so can tie up resources for people who were also struck by the hurricane and who might be trapped in dire situations. Those other people may be seriously injured, they may be trapped, or they may otherwise be in serious danger. If you can keep yourself safe for a while, try to sustain yourself for as long as you can until you truly need help, then call for it. Use a sign in your window that either says "Here, Need Immediate Help" or "Here, No Help Needed," depending on your situation. In either case, rescue crews will know where you are and will be able to prioritize your rescue accordingly based on your level of need. This way, more serious situations are helped first, and those who can sustain themselves for a while longer do not put strain on the rescue crews.

Another time when you might not call for help is when you are in a situation where help cannot do anything, or where help may actually be more dangerous than anything else. For example, many countries have found themselves falling into police states, and they cannot rely on help because that help may actually do more harm than good. In this case, you must seriously assess the emergency and do everything you can to navigate it yourself. If you really cannot, take the person who has endured the emergency and a burner phone, move that person far away from where you are staying, call for help on the burner phone, and leave it with that person. This way, they get the help they need, and you are not at risk of being found and hurt by the police state. While this may seem harsh or you may fear losing that person, it is ultimately better than them suffering without a lack of access to adequate resources and help for their condition.

CONCLUSION

Being in a survival situation can be scary, especially if you do not know what you are getting into. Many people do not realize that you could find yourself inside a serious survival mission within an urban environment, possibly even within your home. Others may be more "traditional" in the sense that you need to escape your home and live in the wilderness for a while until it is safe for you to return.

Knowing how to survive in any situation is important, as it is the first step in getting help and finding your way back to safety. If you fail to survive, you will fail to get the help you need as there will be no more helping you. Many people think the emergency itself is the leading cause of death, but the inability to survive the aftermath also carries a huge death toll. For example, if you find yourself launched into the wilderness after a natural disaster strikes, not knowing how to catch and prepare food or purify water for consumption could lead to your death. These dangers are just as bad as the emergency itself, so you must discover how to properly navigate them and keep yourself safe until you can return to a safer environment.

I hope that through reading *Survival Guide for Beginners 2021,* you feel confident in your ability to navigate any emergency, no matter what it is. Whether you need to survive an urban environment or a wilderness environment, there are many steps you can take to keep yourself alive and safe. Knowing how to take them, and when to take them, will make all the difference.

I strongly encourage you to keep a copy of this book in your G'n'G bag so that if you ever do find yourself in an emergency, you have access to this guide, which will show you exactly how to navigate it. Sometimes, in the face of stress and fear, memory can fail us, so having a hard copy available to go back to is essential to keep you going and keep you safe even in the most dire of times.

Before you go, I also ask that you take a moment to review *Survival Guide for Beginners 2021*. Your honest feedback would be greatly appreciated, and it will help others discover how they, too, can survive any emergency they may face in their lifetimes. This is essential knowledge, so the more people that have it, the better.

Thank you, and best of luck in any situation you may come across. Remember, stay positive, stay focused, get the job done, and keep going. You can do it.

www.ingramcontent.com/pod-product-compliance
Lightning Source LLC
Chambersburg PA
CBHW080459240426
43673CB00005B/235